Walk
With Ease

Your Guide to Walking for Better Health,
Improved Fitness and Less Pain

THIRD EDITION

AN OFFICIAL PUBLICATION OF THE ARTHRITIS FOUNDATION

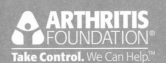

Copyright © 2010, 6th printing.
Library of Congress PCN: 2002100858
ISBN: 978-0-912423-05-0

Published by
The Arthritis Foundation
1330 West Peachtree Street NW, Suite 100
Atlanta, GA 30309

Printed in Canada

The mission of the Arthritis Foundation is to improve lives through
leadership in the prevention, control and cure of arthritis and related
diseases.

Walk
With Ease

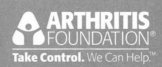

ARTHRITIS
FOUNDATION®
Take Control. We Can Help.™

Table of Contents

Appendix B: Exercises to Help You Warm Up, Stretch, and Cool Down

Appendix C: Resources and References 161

Acknowledgments

The *Walk With Ease* program was originally developed by Terrie Heinrich Rizzo, MAS, Program Director, Health and Fitness Education, Stanford Health Improvement Program, Stanford Center for Research in Disease Prevention. The information and strategies contained throughout the Walk With Ease program are based on research studies and tested programs in the fields of exercise science, behavior modification, and arthritis patient education. In particular, these include research and programs done by the Stanford University Patient Education Research Center; Kate Lorig, RN, DrPH, a nurse and expert in patient education and arthritis self-management; Albert Bandura, PhD, a social psychologist; and Marian Minor, PT, PhD, a physical therapist and expert in exercise and arthritis.

Walk With Ease was based on a pilot program developed by Donna Everix, PT, as part of the San Mateo (California) Arthritis Project (SMAP). The program was developed following the theme of "EASE" (Encourage Arthritis Support and Education).

This third edition of *Walk With Ease* is based on feedback from *Walk With Ease* leaders and participants and a more extensive testing of the program in varying communities. This evaluation and the resulting program modifications were conducted by a team of investigators led by Principal Investigator Leigh F. Callahan, PhD, Thurston Arthritis Research Center, and co-Principal Investigator Mary Altpeter, PhD, MSW, MPA, Institute on Aging, of the University of North Carolina (UNC). Team members contributing to program evaluation and curriculum development also include Jean Goeppinger, PhD, RN; Andrea Meier, PhD, EdM; Britta Schoster, MPH; Thelma Mielenz, PT, PhD, OCS; Margaret Morse, PhD; and Katherine Buysse, BS.

The UNC Chapel Hill team wishes to thank Dr. Peter Blanpied of the University of Rhode Island and Rebecca Fornloff from the Rhode Island region of the Northern and Southern New England chapter of the Arthritis Foundation for sharing their experiences, research findings and program materials from their implementation of the *Walk With Ease* program. The team also wishes to thank the Walk With Ease leaders and participants who have shared their comments about the program that we have used in this edition of the book.

This edition of this publication was partially supported by Cooperative Agreement Number MM 0975-07/07 from the Centers for Disease Control and Prevention and the Association of American Medical Colleges. Its contents are solely the responsibility of the authors and do not necessarily represent the official views of the Centers for Disease Control and Prevention, the Department of Health and Human Services, or the U.S. government.

Chapter 1

Introducing
Walk With Ease

Congratulations on your decision to learn more about walking and its benefits! The *Walk With Ease* program is designed to help you become a knowledgeable, confident arthritis self-manager – that is, a person who can take action to ease arthritis symptoms and maintain your overall fitness and quality of life. *Walk With Ease* may be different from other walking programs you know about, because it offers a structured program that has been tested and proven to benefit those who complete it. This book also offers something that you may not have found before: practical advice on how to walk safely and comfortably, plus lots of strategies to help keep you walking and overcoming challenges that can interfere with an exercise program. Again, congratulations, and we hope you'll enjoy the *Walk With Ease* program and the pleasure of walking that comes with it.

**In this chapter,
you can learn about:**
- Why walking is good for you
- Some basic health considerations
- What the *Walk With Ease* program can offer you
- How the *Walk With Ease* program is designed
- How to use this book and make *Walk With Ease* your own

**You can also
do these activities:**
- Assess your starting point
- Do a self-check to review your progress

Why Walking Is Good for You

Walking is an excellent and simple form of exercise that's good for nearly everyone, from absolute beginners to people who have been physically fit for years. Walking can help you gain all the benefits of exercise, from weight loss to stress control. Walking is easy to do and doesn't require a health club membership, fancy shoes or equipment, or special training. You can do it with friends, loved ones, your pet, or on your own.

There are nearly 50 million people in the U.S. with some form of arthritis. Walking is one of the safest and most beneficial forms of exercise for most people with arthritis and other chronic health conditions. That's why the Arthritis Foundation developed the *Walk With Ease* program. *Walk With Ease* is shown to reduce the pain and discomfort of arthritis and increase balance, strength and walking pace. Either done in a group or on your own, the program can build confidence in your ability to be physically active and improve your overall health. Visit www.arthritis.org/wwe to learn more about the program, to find a group in your area or to access tools, podcasts and online communities to help make your program a success.

Walking, like many other forms of exercise, offers many benefits for your body and spirit. Besides being inexpensive, convenient, and fun, walking has a lot of positive health benefits. Walking is also safer and puts less stress on the body than most other forms of aerobic exercise – the kind that builds stamina and boosts cardiovascular fitness. Walking is an especially good exercise choice if you're older or have been less active.

Walk With Ease participants and group leaders agree. Throughout this book, we're sharing their comments about the benefits of walking and exercise, and specifically, about this program. Who better to share experiences and tips with you than others who know this program?

Some Basic Health Considerations

We've already said that walking is good for almost everyone. Before starting the *Walk With Ease* program, however, it's important to consider some basic questions about your health and health status. It's particularly important to assess your risk if you have certain conditions.

Most people living with arthritis experience joint pain, inflammation, stiffness, and limited mobility. Even so, many can walk for exercise, including you. If you can be on your feet for about 10 minutes to do household chores, shopping, or social activities, then you'll most likely be able to begin a walking program to improve your health. Even if you can't stay on your feet quite that long or can only go a short distance, it's still likely that you'll be able to develop a modified walking routine that will benefit your health and help you feel better.

The American Physical Therapy Association suggests that before you start a walking program you answer these questions:

- Do you have heart trouble?

- Do you have chest pains or pain on your left side (neck, shoulder, or arm) or breathlessness when you are physically active?

Some Things Walking Can Do For You

- Strengthen heart and lungs
- Nourish joints
- Build bones
- Fight osteoporosis
- Burn calories
- Control weight
- Reduce stress
- Improve mood
- Boost energy

- Do you often feel faint or have dizzy spells?

- Do you have high blood pressure?

- Do you have bone or joint problems that could worsen if you are physically active?

- Are you 50 or older and not physically active?

The U.S. Department of Health and Human Services urge people with arthritis to get at least 30 minutes of moderate physical activity at least three days a week. You can get activity in 10-minute intervals.

If you can answer *no to all* of these questions, it gives a general indication that you likely can participate in a physical activity program. If you answered *yes to any* of them, or if you're uncertain, then we recommend that you check with your health care practitioner – physician, nurse practitioner, physician's assistant, occupational therapist, or physical therapist – before you begin this walking program or other forms of physical exercise.

To keep you safe when you walk, be alert for signs of serious danger: severe pain; pressure, tightness, or pain in your chest; nausea; difficulty with breathing; dizziness; severe trembling, or light-headedness. If you experience any of these symptoms, *stop* and call 911.

Other symptoms might indicate that you are working too hard, too soon. If you get cramps or a stitch in your side, a very red face or a very pale one, sweat heavily, feel extremely tired, or have pain in your joints that lasts two hours after you exercised and is greater than you had before, you're overdoing it. Slow down next time.

What the *Walk With Ease* Program Can Offer You

It doesn't matter whether you already walk regularly or you haven't yet started, this book will offer you many suggestions based on proven techniques concerning the right way to build and maintain a walking program. You can participate in the *Walk With Ease* program in a group or do it on your own. In either case, this book will help you:

- Understand the basics about arthritis and the relationship between arthritis, exercise and pain.

- Learn how to exercise safely and comfortably.

- Use methods to make walking fun.

- Make a doable personal walking plan with realistic goals for improved fitness.

- Gather tips, strategies and resources that will help you to "stick with it," even when you don't feel like exercising or when things get in your way.

- Learn about other programs and resources that can help you keep up your walking and even branch out to other exercise and self-management programs that other people with arthritis enjoy.

> *Walk With Ease* was a great social outlet for me because we walked together. It gave me a lift for the day – not only physically, but in my mood too.
>
> – *WALK WITH EASE PARTICIPANT*

Being a Problem Solver

Making changes can be difficult. Throughout this book you'll learn a lot of techniques for solving different kinds of problems and challenges that may prevent you from following your

What's the problem?

What's the cause?

What solutions might work?

weekly walking plan and reaching your walking goals. Living – and exercising – successfully with the pain, stiffness, and fatigue associated with arthritis is achievable if you have a good problem-solving approach. Here are three basic components to successful problem solving.

1. Focus on the problem that's most on your mind. For example, are you worried about getting hurt or having pain? Successful problem solving means being concrete about the problem you most care about and want to solve. To help you set your priorities for what's important to *you*, we include a Starting Point Self-test tool and a walking contract and diary that you can use to keep track of how you're doing.

2. Ask yourself what might be the cause(s) of your problem. Focusing on the exact cause of the problem will help you better understand and solve it. For example, if you have pain while walking, ask yourself questions about the details of that activity. Do you have pain in your feet or in your legs? Do you have pain specifically when you walk for more than 20 minutes or when you walk for shorter intervals?

Maybe the cause of the problem has to do with your feelings or attitudes. Maybe you feel that you don't have time to walk. Ask yourself, is it a lack of time or is it feeling pressured with other responsibilities, or are you feeling that walking isn't a priority or it's boring? By getting to the root of your feelings, you have a better chance of finding solutions to overcome them.

3. Try out different solutions. It's important to be open to exploring and experimenting with a variety of solutions and resources. If you're having a problem with foot pain, maybe a solution is to check your shoes and socks to be sure they're in good condition. Having pain during longer walking stretches may mean that you need to cut back the number of minutes you walk or that you're walking on a surface that's too difficult for you (gravel versus asphalt, for example).

If you feel bored when you walk, you may want to pick a walking buddy to chat with or walk in places where there's lots to look at, like a mall or a zoo. Exploring and trying out different solutions may take time, and it may be frustrating if you experience some failures, but ultimately, learning about and trying out a mix of solutions may achieve the most success. This book, and particularly Chapters 4 and 6, offers many solutions and resources for you to explore.

How the *Walk With Ease* Program is Designed

Walk With Ease was written specifically for people with arthritis, but it can be a practical and useful resource for anyone, whether you have arthritis or not! The contents are based on the latest research in exercise science and behavior change, plus lots of hands-on, helpful suggestions from thousands of people both with and without arthritis who have shared their experiences to help make walking work for you. The *Walk With Ease* program is designed to meet your needs, on your own or with a group.

You don't have to be a regular walker already to start, because *Walk With Ease* is aimed at all fitness levels.

– *WALK WITH EASE PARTICIPANT*

Walk With Ease has four components:

1 Walking

2 Health information

3 Exercises

4 Motivational tips and tools

A very important part of the *Walk With Ease* program is that it is designed for you to adapt to your needs. You make your own walking plan, tailor your exercises and walking times to your needs, and you go at your own pace. The program was specifically designed to be done on your own or by participating with a group of walkers coordinated by a *Walk With Ease* leader. If you are interested in walking with a group, your local Arthritis Foundation office will know if there are *Walk With Ease* programs in your area. (To find an Arthritis Foundation office near you, visit www.arthritis.org or call 800-283-7800.)

Whether you do it on your own or participate with a group, the recommended *Walk With Ease* program model is set up as a six-week program for walking. During that time, we recommend that you work up to walking at least three times a week. The idea is to start at a reasonable amount of time and at a reasonable pace for you and build up to 30 minutes or more of walking each of the days you walk.

Walking is not the only part of the *Walk With Ease* program model. The program also includes three other very important components that will help make this a safe and successful walking program for you: health information, exercises, and motivational tips and tools.

The chart provides an overview of the recommended schedule for the *Walk With Ease* program that includes when to do each of the program components. You may feel that reading three chapters and doing the activities in them may be a lot in the first two weeks, but the chapters are short and the activities will not take much time. You can always skim chapters and then go back and read them more thoroughly

Walk With Ease Recommended Program Schedule

	Weeks						After the 6-week program
	1	2	3	4	5	6	
Read Chapters 1, 2, and 3	X						
Do your Starting Point Self-test (Chapter 1)	X						
Set up your walking plan (Chapters 2 and 3)	X						
Walk! Try to walk at least three days a week.	X	X	X	X	X	X	X
Do the 5-Step Basic Walking Pattern each time you walk (Chapter 5)	X	X	X	X	X	X	X
Follow the FITT principles each time you walk (Chapters 3 and 5)	X	X	X	X	X	X	X
Keep your walking diary each time you walk (Chapter 3)		X	X	X	X	X	X
Read Chapters 4, 5, and 6		X					
Measure your fitness level in weeks 2, 4, and 6, and periodically after the program is over		X		X		X	
Monitor your walking intensity and walking progress (distance, time) (Chapters 3, 4, and 5)		X	X	X	X	X	X
Do a midway assessment of your progress using your walking diary, walking plan, and monitoring techniques (Chapters 3, 4, 5, and 6)				X			
Do your Ending Point Self-test and set up your future walking plan (Chapter 6)						X	
Maintain your walking plan							X

at your leisure. In fact, you can review chapters many times during the six weeks of the program and afterwards. The most important thing is to get started walking.

The chart also lists the activities you can continue after you've completed the six-week program. More information and strategies to keep walking and exercising after the six weeks are over are provided in Chapter 6.

During the first week of doing *Walk With Ease*, we recommend three activities that can help get you off to a good start walking:

During the first week

1 Read chapters 1–3.

2 Do your Starting Point Self-test.

3 Set up your walking plan.

1. Read the first three chapters of this book.

2. Do your Starting Point Self-test.

3. Set up your walking plan.

How to Use This Book: Making *Walk With Ease* Your Own

There is no "one-size-fits-all" program for successful physical activity, including walking. Everyone has different experiences and different types of challenges to overcome. For some, these may be physical problems, for others they may be emotional ones. This book will teach you how to customize a walking program to fit your own needs. With the *Walk With Ease* program, *you* determine your *own* starting point on the road to better fitness and health, and *you* set your *own* goals.

Your starting point is exactly where you are right now. You can work your way up to the recommended walking guidelines. Here are some important things to consider in terms of your mental and physical starting points.

- Are you mentally ready to make walking a part of your everyday life? Are you determined to make time for your walking routine and stick with the goals you set for this program?

- If so, now you need to figure out your physical starting point, that is, the amount of time you currently can walk without discomfort, whether it's for one minute at a time, 10 minutes at a time, 20 minutes at a time, or more.

- If you currently are able to walk for at least 10 minutes, regardless of your speed, you should be able to follow the *Walk With Ease* guidelines just about "as they are laid out." Start at the beginning of the book, and work your way through each chapter. The information presented will help you develop a lasting personal walking routine while you deal with issues of safe exercise, pain management, and motivation that affect nearly everyone.

- However, if you've been inactive; have health problems other than arthritis; or have significant limitations to your hips, knees, or ankles, you may not be able to walk more than a few minutes without discomfort. If so, this book can work for you, too. Just ignore our suggested time guidelines and go at your own pace.

> Feeling better and building friendships are two of the main program incentives of *Walk With Ease*.
>
> – WALK WITH EASE PARTICIPANT

We recommend that you read through all the chapters in order to take full advantage of the information and benefits of the program. Each chapter begins with a summary of the learning points. Each chapter ends with a *Self-check* to help you assess what you've learned and your confidence in doing the program.

Because the chapters are organized in a logical sequence of first getting ready for walking, then beginning your walking, and finally staying motivated and sticking with it, we recommend that you read the chapters in order. Read the information, try out the suggestions, and if necessary, modify them to fit your needs. Go at your own pace. Along the way, ask yourself, "What have I learned about walking and exercise and managing my arthritis?"

Assessing Your Starting Point

To help you figure out your starting point, it's important to determine how arthritis affects your daily life. The *Starting Point Self-test* included in this chapter will help you to consider how common problems associated with arthritis such as pain, fatigue, and physical limitations affect you. The Starting Point Self-test includes scoring instructions.

We encourage you to take the few minutes necessary to complete the Starting Point Self-test. The scoring instructions will let you know where you stand right away. Not only can you learn about your starting point for the beginning of this program, but your score can guide you in highlighting which parts of the book and the *Walk With Ease* program will be particularly important to you.

You can also use the Starting Point Self-test again after the end of six weeks to see whether there have been any improvements. These results can also provide an indication of how you're feeling and how you're managing your arthritis.

Remember

You can do the program at your pace, but we recommend that you:

- Walk at least three days a week, even if you only walk for a short time each time.

- Read the health education information.

- Do the motivational activities including your Starting Point Self-test, your walking plan, and your walking diary (more about these in Chapter 3).

Starting Point Self-test

PAIN

Please circle the number that describes how much physical pain your arthritis has caused during the past week.

0   1   2   3   4   5   6   7   8   9   10
No pain   As bad as it can be

FATIGUE

Please circle the number that describes how much of a problem fatigue has been for you during the past week.

0   1   2   3   4   5   6   7   8   9   10
No problem   A major problem

PHYSICAL LIMITATIONS

The following items are about activities you might do during a typical day. Does your health now *limit* you in these activities? If so, how much? (Circle one number on each line.)

	Not at all	Yes, a little	Yes, a lot
Vigorous activities, such as running, lifting heavy objects, participating in strenuous sports	1	2	3
Moderate activities, such as moving a table, pushing a vacuum cleaner, bowling, or playing golf	1	2	3
Lifting or carrying groceries	1	2	3
Climbing *several* flights of stairs	1	2	3
Climbing *one* flight of stairs	1	2	3
Bending, kneeling, or stooping	1	2	3
Walking *more* than a mile	1	2	3
Walking *several hundred yards*	1	2	3
Walking *one hundred yards*	1	2	3
Bathing or dressing yourself	1	2	3

Add up all the circled numbers and write your total Physical Limitations score in the box:

Starting Point Self-test Scoring Instructions

PAIN

If your score was:

1–3 Pain is probably not your main concern. You may want to make pain management a lower priority for now and focus on other topics in the book.

4–7 Pain is probably an important concern for you. Many of the suggestions in this book will help you to reduce your pain. Information on pain management can be found in Chapters 4 and 6.

8–10 Pain is probably a main problem for you. Tell your health care practitioner that you're experiencing a lot of pain. Medication or a change in medication may help. Many of the suggestions in this book will help you to manage your pain. Information on pain management can be found in Chapters 4 and 6.

FATIGUE

1–3 Fatigue is probably not your main concern. You may want to make fatigue management a lower priority for now and focus on other topics in the book.

4-7 Fatigue is probably an important concern for you. Many of the suggestions in this book will help you to reduce your fatigue. Information on fatigue management can be found in Chapters 4 and 6.

8–10 Fatigue is probably a main problem for you. Tell your health care practitioner if you're experiencing a lot of fatigue. Some medications may cause fatigue. Information on fatigue management can be found in Chapters 4 and 6.

PHYSICAL LIMITATIONS

10–15 You probably don't have many physical limitations. Information in Chapter 5 and the exercises in Appendix B will give you ideas for improving your muscle flexibility, strength, and endurance.

16–22 You have some physical limitations, which can probably be improved if you increase your muscle flexibility, strength, and endurance. Chapter 5 and the exercises in Appendix B will give you ideas for improving your muscle flexibility, strength, and endurance.

23–30 You have many physical limitations. The good news is that consistent exercise will probably help you improve your physical activities. Information in Chapter 5 and the exercises in Appendix B may give you ideas for improving your muscle flexibility, strength, and endurance, but check with your health care practitioner for more suggestions.

Self-check

TEST YOUR KNOWLEDGE
Circle either "yes" or "no" for each of the following statements:

Yes	No	I can name at least three reasons why walking is good for people.
Yes	No	I know the key health questions to ask before starting a walking program.
Yes	No	I can name the four components of the *Walk With Ease* Program.
Yes	No	I understand why assessing my starting point for the *Walk With Ease* program can be useful to me.

RATE YOUR CONFIDENCE LEVEL
On a scale of 0 to 10 with "0" being not confident at all and "10" being totally confident, circle the number that represents how confident you are about the following things.

I feel confident that walking will be beneficial for me.

0	1	2	3	4	5	6	7	8	9	10

Not confident at all   Totally confident

I feel confident that I can use my Starting Point Self-test to adapt the *Walk With Ease* program to fit my needs.

0	1	2	3	4	5	6	7	8	9	10

Not confident at all   Totally confident

NEXT STEPS
Could you answer yes to the statements above? Is your confidence level 7 or more? If so, congratulations! You're ready to move on.

Each of the statements refers to a section of this chapter. If you answered no to any of them, you may wish to go back and review that section. If your confidence is low, review the sections you're not sure about. You can also share questions or concerns with your friends who have arthritis and walk or with your health care practitioner. If you're in a *Walk With Ease* group program, we recommend that you share your questions or concerns with your group leader and fellow participants.

Chapter 2

Know the Basic Facts About Arthritis and Exercise

Arthritis Basics

More than 50 million Americans have been diagnosed with arthritis, and nearly 1 in 10 say arthritis limits their daily activities. One in five people in the United States is affected by arthritis, and almost two-thirds of these people are younger than age 65.

The word arthritis literally means "inflammation of the joints," but that's a little misleading – not all forms of arthritis involve inflammation. Arthritis is a term used for more than 100 medical conditions. In this book we will focus on three of the more common ones, osteoarthritis, rheumatoid arthritis and fibromyalgia. Depending on which condition you have, muscles, connective tissues, bones or other body organs may be affected. In general, arthritis and related conditions cause pain in and around joints and make it hard to move.

In this chapter, you can learn about:
- Arthritis basics
- Osteoarthritis, rheumatoid arthritis, and fibromyalgia
- Exercise and arthritis
- What kinds of exercise to do and how much
- Exercise dos and don'ts
- Additional questions about exercise and modifications

And you can do this activity:
- Do a self-check to review your progress

Specific causes are known for some forms of arthritis but not for most. Because there are so many types of arthritis, there are likely to be many different causes. Scientists currently are studying the roles of three major factors, (1) how you live, (2) what happens to your body during your life, and (3) genetic factors you inherit from your parents. They have identified two factors that increase your chances for developing arthritis that you can do something about, overweight and injury to your joints.

One in five people in the U.S. is affected by arthritis.

People who are overweight are more likely to have some form of arthritis, including gout (especially men) and osteoarthritis of the knees and possibly hips. How much of a factor is being overweight? For some forms, apparently it makes quite a difference. For example, research shows that overweight middle-age women who lose 11 pounds or more over 10 years cut their risk for developing knee arthritis in half.

An injury that occurs to a joint or connective tissue increases the risk for some types of musculoskeletal conditions, such as tendonitis, bursitis, carpal tunnel syndrome, and osteoarthritis of the knees and spine. These types of injuries can be caused by accidental damage or repetitive overuse, including sports-related injuries, accidents, or job-related repetitive movements, such as repetitive deep knee-bending, lifting, reaching, or typing.

Basic Facts About Osteoarthritis, Rheumatoid Arthritis and Fibromyalgia

Osteoarthritis

Osteoarthritis is the most common form of arthritis, and it now affects more than 27 million people in the U.S. This number is expected to grow significantly as the "baby boomer" population ages. Also sometimes known as degenerative joint disease, there are two types of osteoarthritis, primary and secondary. Primary osteoarthritis involves gradual, degenerative wear-and-tear of joint cartilage, and there is no known cause for this type. Secondary osteoarthritis involves degenerative changes of the cartilage related to injury, genetics, obesity, and other causes.

Osteoarthritis commonly affects the knees, hips, fingers, neck, and lower back. Joint discomfort varies from person to person and can range from mild to severe. Most people with osteoarthritis will not experience severe disability or joint deformity and can manage it by using a variety of strategies, including medicines and pain-management techniques. Recent advances in joint replacement have helped people with severe osteoarthritis of the hips or knees.

What about exercise for people with osteoarthritis? Years ago, they were advised to stay off affected joints, but not anymore. Treatment now emphasizes the importance of exercise, and research supports it. We now know that cartilage needs joint motion to stay healthy, because the motion of exercise both delivers nourishment to the joints and gets rid of waste products. Joint cartilage actually deteriorates if a joint is not moved regularly.

If you have osteoarthritis, follow the general exercise dos and don'ts listed in this chapter. Additionally, keep the following points in mind.

KEY POINTS ABOUT OSTEOARTHRITIS

Joints. All joints, especially those with osteoarthritis, need to be moved regularly and taken through their full range of motion several times a day to maintain flexibility and take care of cartilage. Observe safety precautions, but avoid babying joints with osteoarthritis.

Overloaded joints. If you have osteoarthritis in your hips or knees, avoid types of exercise that overload these joints, such as climbing or very fast walking. Also, after you exercise try to rest off your feet for as much as an hour, if you can, to give cartilage time to decompress.

Precautions for artificial joints. If you have had a joint replaced, consult your health care practitioner before attempting any stretching or strengthening exercises for that part of your body. When engaging in aerobic exercise like walking, remember that certain precautions apply to artificial hips and knees, and you need to respect these if you want the joint to last as long as possible.

Moderate activity. Just as too much rest is bad for joints with osteoarthritis, so is too much activity. If joints are continually compressed (as the hips and knees are by long periods of standing), the cartilage can't expand and soak up nutrients and fluid. Therefore, it is important to avoid long periods of compression, and to alternate activity and rest throughout the day.

Exercise and rest. It is very important for you to strike a balance between getting enough exercise and getting enough rest. How much is too much? Follow the two-hour pain rule: Your goal is to exercise so that pain is not worse two hours after you exercise than before you started. If you do too much, cut back the next time to a point that is comfortable. Adjust until you find a level that works for you.

Good shoes and posture. Always practice good posture and wear supportive shoes. Both of these will help protect cartilage and reduce joint pain. Chapters 3 and 5 provide additional information about shoes and good posture.

Strengthening exercises. Be sure to do strengthening exercises. Toned muscles with good endurance help support joints. Key muscle groups to strengthen generally include the muscles that help support the hips, knees, and ankles. See recommended exercises in Appendix B.

Aquatic exercise. Aquatic or water exercise can be very helpful along with a walking program when you have painful joints, because the buoyancy of the water helps support them, making it easier to move.

Body weight. It is extremely important for you to keep your body weight under control. Too much extra weight speeds up damage to weight-bearing joints. Even ten or twenty extra pounds multiplies the force absorbed by your feet, knees, hips and back, not only when you're exercising, but also when you're just going about your daily activities.

Rheumatoid Arthritis

Rheumatoid arthritis is a systemic autoimmune disease – that is, one that affects all of the body because the immune system, which is responsible for fighting infections, instead attacks the body's own tissues. This causes an inflammation of the lining of the joints, and it can affect internal organs. About 1.3 million people in the United States have rheumatoid arthritis.

Rheumatoid arthritis typically affects many different joints throughout the body, usually symmetrically – that is, the same joints on both sides of the body. This is very different from osteoarthritis, which usually affects only a few specific joints and often is one-sided. Joints that may be affected by rheumatoid arthritis include the hands (except for the joints closest to the fingernails), thumbs, wrists, elbows, shoulders, neck, and jaw, as well as the hips, knees, ankles, and feet. Along with joint problems, rheumatoid arthritis can cause generalized fatigue, decreased appetite, and weight loss.

With rheumatoid arthritis, it is typical to see periods of inflammation, called exacerbations or flares, followed by periods when symptoms are less severe, which vary from individual to individual. Symptoms of a flare can include joint swelling, redness, warmth, pain, tenderness, fatigue, morning stiffness, muscle aches, and a feeling of being sick.

There is no cure for rheumatoid arthritis, and the exact cause is unknown. New drugs are allowing people who have it to lead much healthier and more comfortable lives, so early diagnosis and treatment are even more important. Getting the proper balance between exercise and rest, especially during flares, is also important. When a joint is hot, painful, and swollen, resting helps reduce inflammation, which is good. However, with too much rest, muscles lose strength, ligaments and tendons become less strong, and bones get softer. Research now recommends various forms of exercise for people with rheumatoid arthritis. If you have rheumatoid arthritis, keep the following points in mind.

KEY POINTS ABOUT RHEUMATOID ARTHRITIS

Flares. When you have flares, rest as needed, but remember that rest does not mean stopping all activities. Be sure to continue doing very gentle movements. These should include gentle range-of-motion exercises to help maintain joint mobility. Your health care practitioner can guide you.

Aquatic exercise. Aquatic or water exercise can usually be continued during flares, since the buoyancy of the water helps support joints, making movement easier.

Low-impact exercise. During periods when your symptoms are under control, doing a low-impact weight-bearing activity like walking is important for your overall health. Discuss specific recommendations with your health care practitioner, including any restrictions or modifications for your particular condition. When you have flares, cut back as necessary, but gradually work back up to a full program again as soon as you can.

Flexibility and strengthening exercises. Additionally, when you aren't having a flare, you should do regular flexibility and strengthening exercises to maintain the range of motion and strength of supporting muscles necessary for everyday activities. It is important that your flexibility and strength exercises be carefully designed for your specific needs. Knowing which muscles need to be strengthened and how to perform the exercises without stressing your joints is important. Do not engage in strengthening exercises before talking to your health care practitioner about appropriate recommendations.

Posture and joint motion. Always pay careful attention to using your joints appropriately when exercising. Maintaining good posture and joint motion during exercise helps ease joint pain and avoid tightness.

Maintaining mobility. You may not feel like exercising, especially during flares. Remember that movement is important for you to prevent loss of mobility. Be sure your exercise is appropriate, and be sure to do it!

Fibromyalgia

Fibromyalgia is another common arthritis-related condition. The name means pain in the muscles and fibrous connective tissues (the ligaments and tendons). Fibromyalgia affects about 2 percent of the U.S. population. Fibromyalgia is not actually a joint condition, but a syndrome with a set of signs and symptoms, including:

- moderate to severe fatigue or lack of energy

- decreased endurance for exercise

- sleep disturbances

- headaches

- widespread muscle aches

- "tender points" in specific body locations

Other symptoms can include tingling in the face or extremities (hands, arms, feet, or legs), abdominal pain or bloating, alternating constipation and diarrhea, urinary urgency, and skin sensitivity. Pain often varies according to time of day, activity level, sleep patterns, stress, and weather. Most people with this condition say that some degree of pain is always present, and often the aches and discomfort feel like a persistent flu.

Recent research has shown that individualized exercise at the appropriate intensity (low and moderate) is a very important part of treatment for people with fibromyalgia. If you have fibromyalgia, here are points to remember.

KEY POINTS ABOUT FIBROMYALGIA

A specific combination of exercises can be an important part of your treatment program by helping you reduce muscle tension, decrease pain, and aid relaxation. This combination includes:

- regularly participating in low-intensity aerobic activity to improve conditioning and maintain good circulation (all great reasons to walk!)

- carefully performing stretching exercises before and after your aerobic activity to reduce the likelihood of muscle or joint strains and to maintain good range of motion

- carefully observing safety recommendations for exercise in general, especially if you're doing strengthening exercises, to avoid the possibility of minor injuries such as muscle pulls or joint strains

Start slowly! Be aware that fibromyalgia symptoms often get worse – not better – with vigorous exercise, so it is important that you always start slowly, do only low- to moderate-intensity exercise, and avoid fast movements or high impact.

You may not feel like exercising when you're tired or in pain, but remember that exercise is an important part of your treatment. See Chapter 4 for strategies to help manage pain and stay motivated.

Other Arthritis-Related Conditions

Other conditions in the general family of arthritis and related rheumatic disorders include gout, ankylosing spondylitis, systemic lupus erythematosus (lupus), polymyalgia rheumatica, bursitis, tendinitis, carpal tunnel syndrome, scleroderma, Raynaud's phenomenon, and psoriatic arthritis, among many others. For information about these or the many other forms of arthritis, talk with your health care practitioner or contact the Arthritis Foundation.

The Arthritis Foundation has a series of books, *Good Living with Osteoarthritis*, *Good Living with Rheumatoid Arthritis*, and *Good Living with Fibromyalgia*, designed to help people with these conditions. Each book focuses on the specific disease, offering clear explanations of causes and symptoms, diagnostic tests, drugs and surgical therapies, alternative therapies, and self-management techniques, including detailed stretching exercises. Learn more about these and other Arthritis Foundation books in Appendix C.

Exercise and Arthritis

The value of exercise and physical activity in improving your general health, reducing risks, and fighting arthritis symptoms absolutely cannot be overstated. The benefits received from regular exercise have been documented by hundreds of studies. People who are physically active are healthier, feel better, and

> Some people think that people with arthritis are crippled and should not move. I really think that they should be informed that exercise is good for everyone – especially people with arthritis.
>
> *– WALK WITH EASE PARTICIPANT*

live longer than people who are inactive. But regardless of all these general health benefits, many people still believe the myth that exercise is not good for people with arthritis. They are afraid that physical activity will damage their joints and make their arthritis worse.

What Can Exercise Do For You?

Regular exercise (like walking) can help reduce:

- anxiety
- blood pressure
- blood triglycerides and glucose (sugars)
- body fat percentage
- bone loss
- constipation
- depression
- falls and fractures
- frailty and disability of older people
- resting heart rate
- risk of heart attack
- social isolation
- stress

This is wrong! Research studies support the fact that most people with arthritis can safely get all the benefits of exercise without increasing damage or worsening symptoms. These studies show that for most people with arthritis, appropriate regular exercise leads to better flexibility, strength, and endurance, and to less pain, fatigue, and depression.

What Kinds of Exercise and How Much?

A regular exercise program should include three types of exercise:

- flexibility (also known as stretching or range-of-motion)

- strengthening (also known as resistance)

- cardiovascular (also known as aerobic or endurance)

These are important for everyone, and especially for people with arthritis, because each type of exercise plays a role in improving your overall health and fitness, as well as reducing arthritis-related disability and pain.

Flexibility Exercises

Being able to move your joints all the ways they can safely bend – that is, through your whole range-of-motion – increases your flexibility. Losing range-of-motion can reduce your ability to do the basic, everyday activities of living – for example, simple things like reaching up to kitchen cabinets or bending down to pick up something off the floor.

Maintaining range-of-motion is therefore crucial for your quality of life, so flexibility exercises are the foundation of most therapeutic exercise programs for people with arthritis.

Here are five important tips about flexibility exercises:

1. To keep joints mobile and to improve function, flexibility exercises should be done gently and smoothly for 10 to 15 minutes a day (usually every day and working up to 15 minutes a day).

2. Flexibility exercises also are important to do before and after recreational or fitness activities, because stretched muscles and joints help you maintain balance, avoid falls, and prevent injuries.

3. You should do a few easy but important stretches before and after you walk. These are described more fully in Chapter 5 and Appendix B. When you can do 15 minutes of continuous flexibility movements daily, you will have the motion and endurance needed to include strengthening exercises and aerobic exercises into your program.

4. If you've been inactive for some time, or have pain or stiffness that interferes with daily activities, start your exercise program by building a routine of general flexibility exercises. For suggested exercises, talk with your health care practitioner.

5. Another great source of exercise guidance for you if you have arthritis and have not exercised in a while is the Arthritis Foundation Exercise Program, which can be

taken in a class format or at home using the *Take Control With Exercise DVD* or video. Visit www.arthritis.org; see Appendix C for more details).

Strengthening Exercises

Muscle strength is important for lessening the stress on your joints. Stronger muscles help absorb shock and protect your joints from injury. Stronger muscles also help you maintain the strength necessary to perform such everyday tasks as climbing stairs, gardening, or picking up bags of groceries. These exercises use weight or resistance from some source – sometimes your own body – to make your muscles stronger.

Strengthening exercises need only be done three times a week and not on consecutive days, unless your health care practitioner advises otherwise. If your arthritis is not particularly limiting, you probably can do basic strengthening exercises safely by following recommended rules for proper techniques and safety. Especially remember to start slowly and avoid doing too much, too soon.

However, if you're older or if you have been very inactive or if you have rheumatoid arthritis or another condition with limitations, it is important that your strength program be carefully designed for your specific needs. Knowing which muscles need to be strengthened and how to perform the exercises without stressing your joints are key elements in a successful program. Before you do strengthening exercises, it's a good idea to talk to your health care practitioner for appropriate recommendations. (See Appendix B.)

Cardiovascular Exercises

The purpose of cardiovascular exercise is to make your heart, lungs, blood vessels, and muscles work better. These exercises also help to:

- improve your stamina

- strengthen your bones

- improve your sleep

- control your weight

- reduce stress, depression, and anxiety

- relieve pain and stiffness

- improve blood circulation throughout your body

- release a set of hormones called endorphins, which actually diminish the perception of pain

Contrary to what many people think, aerobic or cardiovascular exercise does not have to be really strenuous. Good news from recent research is that moderate physical activity produces the same health benefits as strenuous activities do, with far less risk of injury. Experts in exercise and arthritis have made specific recommendations for a minimum level of cardiovascular exercise: Accumulate at least 30 minutes of moderate-intensity physical activity or exercise on at least 5 days a week, for a total of 2.5 hours per week.

The best forms of aerobic or cardiovascular exercise for people with arthritis include walking; swimming; aquatic exercise; cycling; low-impact aerobic dancing; and exercising on equipment such as treadmills, ski machines, or stationary bicycles. Everyday activities work, too – raking leaves, walking the dog, mowing the lawn, or going out dancing, for example. Note that all of these involve continuous, repetitive movements of your large muscles. Jogging and running also are aerobic, but these produce more strain on the joints.

But What Is "Moderate-Intensity Physical Activity"?

At a moderate level, you should feel as if your body is working, but you should still be able to talk fairly normally and carry on at a comfortable pace. Getting at least 30 minutes of moderate activity on three or more days of the week may sound like a lot, especially in the beginning, but don't worry. The idea is to do what you can do now, and build gradually. (See Chapter 5 for more information about exercise intensity.)

The walking plan in *Walk With Ease* is designed to help you build up to that recommended level of activity. However, even if you never are able to do all 30 minutes at a time, don't worry! Recent research has also shown that 30 minutes of moderate physical activity accumulated in three 10-minute bouts over the course of the day has the same health benefits as one continuous 30-minute session. This book will help you build your program to the longest segments that are manageable for you. For example, to get your total of 30 minutes, you could rake leaves for 10 minutes, later take a 10-minute walk, and then wash your car for 10 minutes.

> Try to accumulate at least 30 minutes of moderate-intensity physical activity or exercise on at least 5 days a week.

Exercise Dos and Don'ts

Here are some basic tips for what to do and not do as you follow the *Walk With Ease* program.

- **DO** build a program that includes the three different kinds of exercise: flexibility, strengthening, and cardiovascular.

- **DO** walk when you have the least pain and stiffness.

- **DO** walk when you're not tired.

- **DO** walk when your medicine (if you're taking any) is having its greatest effect.

- **DO** always include a warm-up and a cool-down (discussed in Chapter 5) whenever you walk.

- **DO** start at your own ability level, move slowly and gently, and progress gradually.

- **DO** avoid becoming chilled or overheated when walking.

- **DO** use heat, cold, and other strategies to minimize pain. (Discussed in Chapter 4)

- **DO** use aids, like walking sticks or canes, if they help.

- **DO** expect that walking may cause some discomfort.

- **DON'T** do too much, too soon. Start slowly and gradually.

- **DON'T** hold your breath when doing anything! Remember, keep breathing.

- **DON'T** take extra medicine before walking to relieve or prevent joint or muscle pain unless prescribed by your health care practitioner.

- **DON'T** walk so fast or far that you have more pain two hours after you finish than before you started (the 2-Hour Pain Rule).

More Questions About Exercising Safely

If you have additional questions related to exercise for your type of arthritis or a related condition, talk with your health care practitioner. Take this book along and discuss what you should do. Be sure to discuss the best level of intensity and length of time for your walks. Also, talk about any changes you might need to make to accommodate any special needs you have. With adaptations as needed, most people with arthritis can develop a successful exercise program that includes walking.

Remember

The evidence concerning exercise and arthritis is loud and clear:

- Your overall program should include three basic kinds of exercise: flexibility, strengthening, and cardiovascular exercises.

- You will not cause damage to yourself with appropriate exercise.

- You can cause damage to yourself by not exercising!

Self-check

TEST YOUR KNOWLEDGE
Circle either "yes" or "no" for each of the following statements:

Yes	No	I can name three basic facts about arthritis and exercise.
Yes	No	I can explain what osteoarthritis, rheumatoid arthritis and fibromyalgia mean.
Yes	No	I know the three main types of regular exercise that I should do and how often I should do them.

RATE YOUR CONFIDENCE LEVEL
On a scale of 0 to 10 with "0" being not confident at all and "10" being totally confident, circle the number that represents how confident you are about the following things.

I feel confident that I can apply the general tips about exercise and arthritis to my walking program.

0	1	2	3	4	5	6	7	8	9	10
Not confident at all   Totally confident

I feel confident that I will not cause damage to myself with exercise.

0	1	2	3	4	5	6	7	8	9	10
Not confident at all   Totally confident

I feel confident that I can walk and exercise at my own pace, building up to at least 30 minutes on 3 days or more per week.

0	1	2	3	4	5	6	7	8	9	10
Not confident at all   Totally confident

NEXT STEPS
Could you answer yes to the statements above? Is your confidence level 7 or more? If so, congratulations! You are ready to move on.

Each of the statements refers to a section of this chapter. If you answered no to any of them, you may wish to go back and review that section. If your confidence is low, review the sections you're not sure about. You can also share questions or concerns with your friends who have arthritis and walk or with your health care practitioner. If you're in a *Walk With Ease* group program, we recommend that you share your questions or concerns with your group leader and fellow participants.

Chapter 3

Preparing to
Walk With Ease

Walking for exercise isn't complicated – you start a walking program by starting to walk! However, if you're like most people who begin an exercise program, starting is only half the battle. Good intentions usually aren't enough to keep people going for long.

After just six months, nearly half of all those who start exercising have dropped out, and another third will have quit by the end of the first year. Real long-term success at sticking with an exercise program almost always takes more than simply having good intentions; it takes some knowledge, some preparation, some basic information about exercise, and a plan.

**In this chapter,
you can learn about:**
- Choosing shoes, socks and clothes to keep you comfortable
- Planning your walking program so that it's "FITT"
- Choosing where to walk
- Developing a walking plan

**You can also
do these activities:**
- Make your walking plan
- Start your walking diary
- Do a self-check to review your progress

> It's really important to keep your shoes up to date. Don't take a chance with your shoes. Make sure they fit well. You will notice the difference.
>
> *– WALK WITH EASE PARTICIPANT*

Choosing the Right Shoes, Socks and Clothes

One of the greatest things about walking is that you don't need a lot of equipment. All you really need are three things: a pair of sturdy, comfortable shoes, a pair of socks that have good cushioning, and comfortable clothing.

Shoes

Well-fitting, comfortable shoes are crucial for walking. Because the biomechanics – efficient body movements – of walking are different from those for other activities, you shouldn't use just any athletic-type shoes you happen to have around. To provide the best support and help prevent injuries, you should get a good pair of shoes that are comfortable for walking.

What's good when it comes to picking out shoes? See the box on the next page for a handy checklist based on recommendations from the American Physical Therapy Association (www.apta.org). Your shoes should provide good support, be comfortable, and not make your feet hurt. Don't think that the most expensive shoe is the best one for you. Good walking shoes are available in a lot of stores at a variety of prices. Consumers Union (publishers of *Consumer Reports*, probably available at your local library) and other groups do annual evaluations of walking shoes. These can give you some good ideas, but use those ratings only as a guide. Every shoe and every foot is different. Compare prices and do a little research to find the right pair.

Shoe Checklist

Look for these things when you're deciding what shoes to wear for walking:

Insole: The insole should match the arch of your foot.

Sole: The sole should be made from a foam material for cushioning and it should bend at the forefoot rather than the midfoot.

Heel: The heel should be made from a foam material to provide shock absorption.

Heel grip: The heel grip should hold the heel snugly in place. A padded cuff at the top opening may provide a firmer grip and cause less friction on the skin.

Shoe material: Breathable materials such as leather and cotton canvas are preferable to synthetics or plastic.

Toe box: The toe box should provide plenty of wiggle room for the toes in both depth and width.

Proper fit: Always try on both shoes with the same type of socks you will be wearing when walking. If you use any orthotic supports, fit them in the shoes before deciding. Shoes should fit you comfortably, have a snug heel fit so your heel doesn't slip, and have a roomy toe box – enough room to allow your toes to spread out. There should be a thumb's width between the end of your longest toe and the end of the shoe. Shop for shoes at the end of the day, when your feet tend to be at their largest size.

Closures: Shoes with laces let you adjust as needed and give more support than slip-on shoes. If you have problems tying laces, consider Velcro closures or elastic shoelaces.

When should you replace your shoes? Probably sooner than you think – most people wait too long. Shoes might look great from the outside for years, but the insides will lose at least a third of their ability to support and absorb shock and the soles will begin to deteriorate after about 500 miles to 600 miles of walking. That's not as much as it might seem. For example, a walker who takes 30-minute walks three times a week will need replacement shoes after about 9 to 12 months. And the insoles probably will need replacement even sooner – usually every couple of months for people who walk regularly – this is important for shock absorption. Don't continue to wear shoes or insoles when they're worn out. Your body will feel the negative effects.

Socks

Next to your shoes, socks are your feet's best friends. Having the right socks will keep your feet cool and dry, as well as properly cushioned when you walk. As with shoes, don't wear just any socks when you walk or do any other form of exercise. See the Sock Checklist on the opposite page for some recommendations about good walking socks.

Clothes

With the right clothes, you should be able to walk all seasons of the year. Clothes should be comfortable, simple, and efficient. Choices range from simple loose-fitting T-shirts and shorts or sweat suits, to stretch-type walking shorts and tights. See the Clothes Checklist for recommendations.

Sock Checklist

Pick the right sock material. Many walkers prefer padded socks made from a blend of acrylic fiber and cotton or wool. The acrylic wicks away perspiration from your skin, and the cotton or wool then absorbs it, so your feet stay drier and more comfortable.

Wear two. For some blister-prone people, wearing two pairs of socks can eliminate rubbing.

Get the proper fit. Look for snug-fitting socks with as few seams as possible to avoid chafing.

Watch for wear. If your socks wear through in the toes, the problem is your shoes. Either the shoes are too short, or your foot is sliding forward with each step

Match sock fit with shoe fit. Take your walking socks when you go to purchase your shoes to help get a better fit.

Dress as warmly as necessary for the weather. Think layers. The most efficient way to maintain a comfortable body temperature is by wearing layers of clothing. It helps you maintain a constant temperature because the air between layers captures your body heat. If you get too hot, you can remove items of clothing one layer at a time. It is better to start out with too many clothes and remove layers as you go than to be underdressed and too cool to continue walking. This also helps you adjust to your surroundings if part of your walk is outdoors and part indoors.

Clothes Checklist

Choose clothes that allow free movement.
Clothing should allow you to move through the full range of your walking stride without binding, restricting movement, or pulling. Pants or shorts should fit comfortably in the waist and not bind in the leg or crotch.

Select lightweight, absorbent material. Clothing made of cotton is always comfortable and absorbs perspiration. Garments with Supplex®, polypropylene, and fleece are lightweight, draw moisture away from your skin, and provide insulation against the wind.

Wear the right undergarments. Women should wear a comfortable bra that provides good support or a sports bra. If you've never worn a sports bra, try one. You might like the support.

Wear bright or reflective clothing. It is a good idea to wear reflective clothing or a vest with reflectors when you're walking outdoors, even in daylight hours, so that oncoming cars and trucks can see you.

Three layers are generally recommended.

- The inner layer allows for absorption of moisture from the skin and, depending on the material, may pass moisture on to the next layer. Women should always wear a cotton-blend bra, which is usually enough of an inner layer during warmer months.

- The middle layer provides warmth and some protection from wind and cold.

- The outer layer is necessary when walking in colder weather. It should be resistant to wind and rain, allow sweat to evaporate, and, in coldest temperatures, trap air to keep you warm. Nylon is a good material to wear for this layer. A zip or pullover jacket (with or without a hood) will provide protection and also is lightweight. In the coldest months, a hat (and possibly a face mask) should be worn to maintain body heat and protect your face against wind and cold. Mittens or gloves should be worn to keep hands warm.

A mile is about 2,000 steps – more if you have a short stride, or less if you have a long stride.

Other Helpful Things You Might Use

Although we've said that the only things you really need to get you walking are the right shoes, socks, and clothing, here are a few other things you might consider using that can make your walking safer and more enjoyable:

- A watch with second hand or a stopwatch to measure how many minutes of walking you're doing.

- A pedometer to measure how many steps you've walked. Generally, one mile is about 2,000 average steps. If you have a shorter stride, one mile is about 2,400 steps, and for a longer one, it's about 1,900 steps.

- A walking stick or cane for balance and joint support, if recommended by your health care practitioner.

- A fanny pack or small purse to carry miscellaneous items like keys, identification, cell phone, money, and a plastic water bottle.

- A hat or visor on sunny days to protect your face from the sun; on cold days, a warm hat or ear muffs to help you keep warm.

- Sunglasses to reduce eyestrain and eye damage.

Sun protection is important. The Skin Cancer Foundation recommends using sunscreen for all outdoor activities all year round. Put sunscreen on all exposed body parts (don't forget your neck and ears).

Planning Your Program of FITT Exercise

F-I-T-T are the initials we use for the principles of what is necessary to get the most benefit from your exercise. FITT stands for Frequency (how often you exercise), Intensity (how hard), Time (duration – how long), and Type (what kind). If you're doing the *Walk With Ease* program on your own, you can feel confident about building a successful walking program by following the FITT recommendations, which were designed by exercise experts from the American College of Sports Medicine to help people become fitter, healthier, and more pain-free.

F for Frequency

Frequency refers to how often you walk or do another physical activity. The guidelines for people with arthritis recommend at least 30 minutes of walking on at least 5 days a week. If you choose, walking more often is fine, up to all seven days each week, especially if you're walking for short time segments.

When you're able to go for walks of 30 minutes or longer, however, taking days off gives your body a chance to rest and adapt. Try to space your sessions throughout the week. For example, if you're walking and exercising four days a week, you might schedule your walks for Monday, Wednesday, Friday, and Sunday, rather than Monday, Tuesday, Wednesday, and Thursday, followed by three days off. If you walk five days per week, schedule a day off every two or three days. For example, you might walk on Tuesday, Wednesday, Thursday, Saturday, and Sunday. On days when you don't walk, continue to do your flexibility exercises (more about these in Chapter 5). You should do strengthening exercises three to four times a week.

I for Intensity

Intensity refers to how much you're exerting yourself, that is, how hard you're working. The new guidelines for a physical activity like walking recommend exertion at low-to-moderate intensity. What does "low-to-moderate" mean? Use your body's effort as a guideline: At low-to-moderate intensity, you will be working hard enough to feel some changes in your body, such as increased breathing, heart rate, or muscle use, but not so much that you become out of breath or feel that it's hard to keep up.

If exercise is too high in intensity (what you'd describe as hard to very hard), it most likely is too fast or too challenging for your level of fitness right now. Very high intensity exercise almost always causes discomfort, certainly increases your risk of injury, and you're much more likely to stop doing it regularly.

Measuring your intensity as you exercise helps you monitor yourself for safety, so that you don't overdo it. It also helps you keep track of your progress from week to week. Doing this doesn't have to be complicated. You can give yourself a "talk test" while you're exercising (that is, can you exercise and still talk normally to someone else?) or rate how hard you're exercising on a scale of 1 to 10. For most people these informal measures work just fine, especially in the beginning. Taking your pulse is another way to measure yourself. Chapter 5 provides complete guidelines on all of these techniques.

T for Time

Time (duration) refers to how many minutes you spend walking or doing another physical activity. How much time should you spend walking? The new guidelines recommend at least 30 minutes of cardiovascular exercise at least 5 times a week.

Here's a very important tip about your walking time. If 30 minutes at a time is too much for you to start with, remember that your 30 minutes don't have to be done all at once to get health benefits, especially in the beginning. To get 30 minutes of activity on your exercise days, you could walk 30 minutes all at once, or 15 minutes twice a day, or 10 minutes three times a day.

The goal of cardiovascular exercise like walking is to gradually build your endurance and ability to go for a longer time. Begin slowly with short distances or take several short walks a day until you can build up to longer distances and periods of time. As a long-term goal, this walking program will help you build up to at least 30 minutes a session for at least three days a week. However, if pain is a problem, it's ok to stay with shorter segments.

T for Type of Exercise

Different types of physical activities that work different muscle groups contribute to a well-rounded exercise program. The *Walk With Ease* program includes flexibility, stretching, strengthening, and cardiovascular exercises (see Chapter 2 and Appendix B). Combining these types of exercises can help build endurance, flexibility, and overall fitness, if you keep doing them on a regular basis. Remember, to reduce your risk of injury, work at a pace that is comfortable for you, and build up slowly in each type of exercise you do.

Choosing a Good Place to Walk

There are many places to walk that are free and many may be easily accessible.

It's important to choose a place that has a good walking surface. Why? Actually, the walking surface affects the intensity of the exercise you're getting, and it determines the impact – that is, how hard your body is coming down on your feet and joints – and it also interacts with your balance.

If you're doing the *Walk With Ease* program on your own, or if you're walking at other times than when your *Walk With Ease* group meets, it's important to try to choose a walking surface that is suitable for your ability. Consult the table to learn more about how the surface you choose can influence your success.

Impact is a major consideration for many people who have arthritis, particularly in the hips or knees. If you find that you're having pain that you think results from high impact, be sure that you're wearing shoes with insoles that absorb shock and that you're walking on an appropriate, level surface. You may also want to use a walking stick or cane for additional support (see Chapter 4 for suggestions about this). Longer term, keeping your weight at a healthy level can help.

If you find you still can't walk even very short distances without significant joint discomfort in your legs – even after following all precautions and using appropriate pain-management strategies – then you probably should choose a form of cardiovascular exercise that avoids impact – that is, there is no or minimal stress placed on your hips, knees, and feet. Examples include water exercises or a stationary bicycle.

Where Shall We Walk?

Outdoor Areas
- Any neighborhood with sidewalks
- Downtown
- Outdoor shopping strips
- Parks
- School yards and tracks
- Community walking trails
- Cemeteries

Indoor Areas
- Shopping malls
- Convention centers
- Large warehouse stores
- Churches
- Museums
- Your home
- Your office

Developing Your Walking Plan

Now that you've learned what makes for a FITT exercise program and thought about what to wear when you walk and where to walk, it's time to make a plan. Research has shown that people who make plans of action – and write them down and review them each week – have greater success in meeting their goals than people who don't make written plans. There are six principal parts to a walking plan that make it most effective: (1) making a contract with yourself about your walking goals; (2) keeping records of your walking in a diary or on a calendar; (3) using self-measurement tools to check your progress; (4) checking your plan every week; and most importantly, (5) deciding how to reward yourself for sticking to the program, as well as for reaching your goals. Finally, (6) keep going by making a new contract.

This section describes how to do all six steps, and at the end of the chapter you will find some of the tools you can try out as you begin this program. We've also provided an example of how you might fill them out. We'll revisit your walking contract in Chapter 6. Also, there are blank tools in Appendix A that you can write on or photocopy. After the program is finished, you may want to tailor these tools to support you in continuing to walk.

Choosing a Suitable Walking Surface

Level I: Flat, firm surfaces such as school tracks, streets with sidewalks, shopping malls, fitness trails, or quiet neighborhoods. Most people with arthritis and related conditions should walk on Level I surfaces.

- most adaptable for intensity (i.e., exertion from low- to high-intensity is possible)
- least impact to knees and hips
- least challenging to balance

Level II: Some inclines or stairs, somewhat uneven ground such as sand, gravel, or soft earth.

- more challenging in intensity
- greater impact to knees and hips
- more challenging to balance

Level III: Hills, very uneven ground with very loose gravel or stones, or lots of stairs. Most people with arthritis should avoid Level III surfaces when walking as a cardiovascular exercise.

- most challenging in intensity (i.e., the lowest level of exertion is even harder)
- greatest impact to knees and hips
- most difficult for balance

If you're doing the program as part of a *Walk With Ease* group, you can discuss your walking plan with other participants and also hear about their plans. You can be a support to each other in carrying out your respective plans. If you're doing the program on your own, you may want to share your plan with a friend or family member who can support your efforts. Here are the basic steps in developing your plan.

Make a Contract with Yourself

First, think about your goals in doing this program and how long it might take you to accomplish them. Six weeks is a reasonable time commitment to start with, and that's the framework this book uses. What do you want to accomplish? What is reasonable to expect in six weeks?

- If you have been extremely limited in your activities because of pain or disability, your first goal may be to walk five minutes at a time in your own home or around the block each day.

- If you have fallen into inactivity by habit or discomfort, you may be able to start out by walking slowly for 10 minutes at a time, three times a week.

- If you're already active, you may be able to go for longer walks, perhaps for 20 minutes or more at a time, at least three days a week.

Six Parts of a Walking Plan

1 Set goals and make a contract.

2 Keep records.

3 Use self-tests to measure progress.

4 Check your plan every week.

5 Reward yourself!

6 Make a new contract.

Be realistic in your expectations, and consider that achieving long-term goals can be the result of achieving several shorter-term steps. For example, many people can't start off by walking for 30 minutes three days a week (long-term goal), but most people can walk for at least a few minutes to begin with (achievable step). Once you have met your short-term goal, you can set a new one that is more challenging and work on that.

The more specific you can be with your plan, the easier it will be to know when you've accomplished your goals. Here are some steps that will help you be specific.

- Assess yourself honestly. Start with where you are. You may be able to start by walking 10 or 15 minutes at a time three days a week or right now you may only be able to walk a few minutes a day. Either place is fine if it's appropriate for you.

- State exactly how much you will do. Specify as many minutes as you will walk. You may decide to follow the suggested progression chart included in Chapter 5 exactly, or you may decide to walk for less (or more), depending on your level of readiness. When you're thinking about how much time you'll spend each time you walk, don't forget to allow time for your warm-up and cool-down exercises.

- State when you will walk. Again, be specific whether you'll walk before breakfast, during your lunch break, immediately after work, or take an evening walk with the dog.

- State how often you will walk. It usually is best to contract to do something three days a week. If you do more, that's a bonus. All people have days when they don't feel like doing anything or can't, because other commitments get in the way. If you say you will walk three or four days a week, though, you can probably still meet your contract even if there are days when you aren't able to do your walk.

- Look at your contract every day. Once you've designed a plan that you're happy with, write the final contract down and post it where you'll see it every day. The contract can be a great tool for you to help you stay focused and on track with your walking program.

Keep a Walking Diary

Research also shows that keeping records of your weekly activity helps you make and maintain changes in your overall level of physical activity. Some people find that just being able to write down that they've accomplished their daily walking goal is rewarding all by itself. Keeping a diary as part of your walking plan can be simple or elaborate, but it often helps to note what is helping you keep walking, what the challenges are, and how you plan to handle the challenges.

There is a weekly diary at the end of this chapter to help you keep track of how much you walk, so you can keep an eye on your progress. Use the six weeks of this program to experiment – find out what works best for you. Appendix A also contains another copy of the diary for you to use, now, or as you continue walking after the program ends.

Do Some Self-test Measurements

Self-tests can be a great motivator for sticking with the program, because you can see how the program is helping. Self-tests can be very easy to do and not time-consuming. After you read Chapter 1, you probably completed the Starting Point Self-test. You can take it again – and in fact, we recommend that you do an Ending Point Self-test at the end of week six of the program. There's a place to record your Starting Point Self-test and Ending Point Self-test scores in your walking diary. Also, you can measure your fitness level by measuring the amount of time you're able to walk, or the distance you're able to walk, or take a physical measurement such as your heart rate. Chapter 5 has instructions for how to do these three fitness tests. We encourage you to do fitness tests as part of your walking plan, particularly at the beginning, middle, and end of the six-week program. There's a place to record the date and results in your walking diary.

Check your progress regularly! Do some self-test measurements and check your plan.

Check Your Plan Every Week

At the end of each week, take stock of how well your walking program is working. For example, are you feeling less fatigued? Are you enjoying yourself? If you've done a fitness test, do you see changes? Have you managed to do what you planned in your contract?

If you're having difficulty, this is a good time to use "consultants" to help you accomplish your goal. Depending on the problem (motivation, logistics, pain), your consultants may be friends, family, your *Walk With Ease* leader or fellow participants, other exercise leaders, or health care practitioners. Then, as with any plan that may need modifying, make changes if necessary. Decide what worked and what made exercising difficult.

If you've been making notes, look over your diary for ideas about what helps or gets in the way. You may decide to change the place or time you exercise, your exercise partners, your routes, your pain management strategies, or other things that will make your program more enjoyable and successful.

Reward Yourself for Accomplishing Your Goals

It's very important to give yourself rewards as you go along – not necessarily with expensive treats or with junk food, but by incorporating things that are pleasant and meaningful to you. Meeting your goals and sticking with the program is worth celebrating! We recommend that you plan a "midway" reward after you've been walking for three weeks, and another reward at the end of the program.

There are many ways to mix rewards into your walking program. For example, if you enjoy watching TV in the evening, you might put it off until after you've walked. The pleasurable act of watching your favorite program turns into a reward for accomplishing your daily goal. Treats could be anything from a new exercise book to a sunrise walk with a special friend. But also congratulate yourself with that special treat for your completion of your contract – for

What would be a good reward for accomplishing your goals? Write some choices here.

_____

_____

_____

_____

_____

_____

_____

_____

_____

example, the new pair of walking shoes or the celebratory healthy dinner. Think of things that would be pleasurable to you, and plan to give yourself some of these at intervals throughout your contract.

Make a New Contract

At the end of your six-week contract period for the *Walk With Ease* program, assess your progress and make a new contract based on your new (or continuing) goals. In your week 6 diary, we've added questions to help you review all six weeks of your program.

To make a new contract, simply follow the basics for planning outlined in this chapter. Do remember to set a specific time period – six weeks or maybe a little longer – during which you keep an eye on your progress and give yourself small rewards. And at the end of that time, make a new contract. Remember, your aim is to continue with a lifetime of walking!

Self-check

TEST YOUR KNOWLEDGE
Circle either "yes" or "no" for each of the following statements:

Yes	No	I know how to select appropriate equipment for walking, including shoes, socks, clothing and any aids I need.
Yes	No	I can describe the FITT principles of walking.
Yes	No	I understand the components and process for making a realistic and achievable walking plan.

RATE YOUR CONFIDENCE LEVEL
On a scale of 0 to 10 with "0" being not confident at all and "10" being totally confident, circle the number that represents how confident you are about these statements.

I feel confident that I can apply the FITT principles to my walking program.

0   1   2   3   4   5   6   7   8   9   10
Not confident at all   Totally confident

I feel confident that I can use my weekly diary and my contract to set goals and keep track of my progress.

0   1   2   3   4   5   6   7   8   9   10
Not confident at all   Totally confident

I feel confident that I can walk and exercise at my own pace, building up to at least 30 minutes on 3 days or more per week.

0   1   2   3   4   5   6   7   8   9   10
Not confident at all   Totally confident

NEXT STEPS
Could you answer yes to the statements above? Is your confidence level 7 or more? If so, congratulations! You're ready to move on.

Each of the statements refers to a section of this chapter. If you answered no to any of them, you may wish to go back and review that section. If your confidence is low, review the sections you're not sure about. You can also share questions or concerns with your friends who have arthritis and walk or with your health care practitioner. If you're in a *Walk With Ease* group program, we recommend that you share your questions or concerns with your group leader and fellow participants.

Sample Contract

From (date): _January 7, 2008_ To: _February 19, 2008_

I, _____ _Pat Walker_ _____ plan to walk

___3___ days a week

for _30_ minutes a day or _____ (distance),

broken into _____ _2 15-minute_ _____ sessions.

I plan to walk _first thing in the morning and after dinner_

(time of day, e.g., at lunch, after dinner).

I will spend 3 to 5 minutes warming up and

4 to 5 minutes doing warm-up stretches

and 3 to 5 minutes cooling down and

7 to 9 minutes doing cool-down stretches.

When I get halfway through this program (week 3), my reward to myself will be:

Dinner at the new vegetarian restaurant with friends

When I complete this program, my reward to myself will be:

A new backpack

Signature: _Pat Walker_

Sample Walking Diary

Week 1

Goal: ___ total minutes or ___ total distance for the week. How did I do each day?

Sunday _____

Monday *15 minutes morning and evening* _____

Tuesday _____

Wednesday *15 minutes morning, 10 minutes evening* _____

Thursday _____

Friday *No morning, 15 minutes at lunch, 15 minutes after dinner*

Saturday _____

Starting Point Self-test Pain: _6_ Fatigue: _7_ Physical Limitations: _____

What's helping me to keep walking?

My walking buddy, losing 2 pounds, feeling happier _____

_____

_____

What's been a challenge for me to keep walking?

Late from work on Wednesday, bad weather in the morning on Friday, but

I made it up at lunch. _____

_____

What information do I need to help me handle the challenges and where can I get it?

We need to find some nice indoor places to walk when it's bad out.

I need to put my walking schedule on my calendar and treat it like an

important appointment! _____

Contract

From (date): _____To: _____

I, _____ plan to walk

_____ days a week

for _____ minutes a day or _____ (distance),

broken into _____ sessions.

I plan to walk _____

(time of day, e.g., at lunch, after dinner).

I will spend 3 to 5 minutes warming up and

4 to 5 minutes doing warm-up stretches

and 3 to 5 minutes cooling down and

7 to 9 minutes doing cool-down stretches.

When I get halfway through this program (week 3), my reward to myself will be:

When I complete this program, my reward to myself will be:

Signature: _____

Walking Diary

Week 1

Goal: ___ total minutes or ___ total distance for the week. How did I do each day?

Sunday _____

Monday _____

Tuesday _____

Wednesday _____

Thursday _____

Friday _____

Saturday _____

Starting Point Self-test Pain:_____ Fatigue: _____ Physical Limitations: _____

What's helping me to keep walking?

_____

_____

_____

What's been a challenge for me to keep walking?

_____

_____

_____

What information do I need to help me handle the challenges and where can I get it?

_____

_____

_____

Walking Diary

Week 2

Goal: ___ total minutes or ___ total distance for the week. How did I do each day?

Sunday _____

Monday _____

Tuesday _____

Wednesday _____

Thursday _____

Friday _____

Saturday _____

This week I chose this as my fitness measure:

_____

What's helping me to keep walking?

_____

_____

_____

What's been a challenge for me to keep walking?

_____

_____

_____

What information do I need to help me handle the challenges and where can I get it?

_____

_____

_____

Walking Diary

Week 3

Goal: ___ total minutes or ___ total distance for the week. How did I do each day?

Sunday _____

Monday _____

Tuesday _____

Wednesday _____

Thursday _____

Friday _____

Saturday _____

What's helping me to keep walking?

_____

_____

_____

What's been a challenge for me to keep walking?

_____

_____

_____

What information do I need to help me handle the challenges and where can I get it?

_____

_____

_____

Do I remember to reward myself?

_____

Walking Diary

Week 4

Goal: ___ total minutes or ___ total distance for the week. How did I do each day?

Sunday   _____

Monday   _____

Tuesday   _____

Wednesday   _____

Thursday   _____

Friday   _____

Saturday   _____

Now my fitness level is:

_____

What's helping me to keep walking?

_____

_____

_____

What's been a challenge for me to keep walking?

_____

_____

_____

What information do I need to help me handle the challenges and where can I get it?

_____

_____

_____

Walking Diary

Week 5

Goal: ___ total minutes or ___ total distance for the week. How did I do each day?

Sunday _____

Monday _____

Tuesday _____

Wednesday _____

Thursday _____

Friday _____

Saturday _____

What's helping me to keep walking?

_____

_____

_____

What's been a challenge for me to keep walking?

_____

_____

_____

What information do I need to help me handle the challenges and where can I get it?

_____

_____

_____

_____

_____

Walking Diary

Week 6

Goal: ___ total minutes or ___ total distance for the week. How did I do each day?

Sunday _____

Monday _____

Tuesday _____

Wednesday _____

Thursday _____

Friday _____

Saturday _____

Ending Point Self-test Pain:_____ Fatigue: _____ Physical Limitations: _____

Now my fitness level is:

_____

What's helping me to keep walking?

_____

_____

What's been a challenge for me to keep walking?

_____

_____

What information do I need to help me handle the challenges and where can I get it?

_____

_____

Did I remember to reward myself?

_____

Thinking About All Six Weeks

How did I do overall?

_____

_____

_____

_____

_____

_____

What do I want to change?

_____

_____

_____

_____

_____

_____

_____

Other notes:

_____

_____

_____

_____

_____

_____

_____

Chapter 4

Anticipating and Overcoming Barriers

In Chapter 1, we talked about three components that go into successful problem solving that you could apply to your walking program: (1) setting a priority to address the problem you care most about; (2) analyzing the specific cause or causes of the problem; and (3) trying out different solutions. Your walking plan and diary can really help you focus on your goals and what matters most to you by helping you take stock of your progress and challenges. So stick with them! This chapter will also help you solve problems by providing strategies for and tips about anticipating and overcoming physical and mental barriers to walking.

**In this chapter,
you can learn about:**
- What to do if exercise hurts
- Solving other common difficulties

**You can also
do these activities:**
- Do a self-check to review your progress
- Keep your walking diary
- Review your walking plan

What to Do If Exercise Hurts

Most people with arthritis have pain and discomfort. For many, it is the number one concern, and all too often, it becomes a barrier to starting and sticking with an exercise program. Remember, the pain caused by arthritis and related conditions can come from at least three sources:

- **Damaged and/or inflamed joints and other tissues.** This is the pain caused directly by the condition.

- **Weak, tense muscles.** When a joint is damaged, the natural response of the body is to protect the joint by tensing surrounding muscles. Unfortunately, many people have weak muscles that can't take the stress. Additionally, tense muscles themselves cause pain by building up lactic acid.

- **Fear and depression.** When you're upset or depressed, everything seems worse, including pain. Research shows that pain can cause people to be fearful of movement.

It's important to recognize right here at the beginning that exercising may not be pain-free. Exercise itself may include some accompanying discomfort. For many people with arthritis, exercise can be accompanied by temporary discomfort and new feelings in your muscles and around your joints. You may experience any of the following: cramping or fatigue in your muscles while you walk, discomfort in your knees during or after walking, soreness around your ankles, and soreness in your calf or thigh muscles after walking. However, regular physical activity

Regular physical activity plays a big role in managing overall pain by helping protect joints, making supporting muscles stronger, reducing muscular stress, lessening depression and helping you just feel better.

plays a big role in managing overall pain by helping protect joints, making supporting muscles stronger, reducing muscular stress, lessening depression, and helping you just feel better.

Here are some simple techniques to help you manage pain and discomfort so you can keep walking. Some of them focus on physical things you can do for your body, while others focus on changing your mental outlook and attitude. Some are things you can do immediately – today – as you start your walking program, but others are things that might take you a little time to do. Once you've found several you like or find helpful, take a few minutes to think how you will use each one. Then, place some clues in your environment to remind yourself about your pain-management techniques. For example, place some reminder stickers or notes where you will see them – on your bathroom mirror, the dashboard of your car, your computer monitor, or your gym bag. You could also have a friend or family member remind you.

Techniques for Coping with Pain and Discomfort after Exercising

"What can I do today?"

Use heat and/or cold. Both heat and cold can be affordable, effective, and easy-to-use solutions for pain relief. Many people find heat most helpful before exercise and cold most helpful afterward. Try it for yourself, and use either or both as needed. Heating an inflamed joint is ill-advised, however, because the increased blood flow can make the inflammation worse. Never fall asleep while lying on a heating pad or using an ice pack.

Heat produces an increase in blood flow, helps reduce stiffness, has a sedative effect on painful nerve endings, and relaxes aching muscles and joints. Heating pads and warm showers are good sources of heat. Heat treatments should feel soothing and comfortable, not hot. Always look at your skin for any signs of burns right after using a hot pack and for 24 hours after that.

- Take a long, very warm shower when you first wake up to ease morning stiffness or before you exercise.

- Buy a moist heating pad from the drugstore or make your own by putting a wet washcloth in a plastic freezer bag and heating it in the microwave for one minute. Wrap the hot pack in a towel and place it over the affected area for 15 to 20 minutes.

- If you buy an electric heating pad, try to find one that requires that the "on" switch be held down for the pad to heat. Use only the medium and low settings, and never use the medium setting for more than 20 minutes. Of course, stop if you have pain, too much heat, or burning. Follow the directions on the pad for use.

Cold applications also can be effective against pain. Cold can help control inflammation and swelling, relieve pain, and reduce muscle spasm. When applying the cold you will go through several stages. You will first feel the cold, followed a mild stinging/burning, then a brief aching sensation, and finally the area will go numb. You will pass through these sensations over the first 5 to 8 minutes.

Leave the cold pack on for 10 to 15 minutes. It is a good idea to put a damp cloth between your skin and the pack. Also, allow at least two hours between treatments. Ice packs are best applied with an elastic wrap to provide some compression. You should only use about two-thirds of the available stretch in the wrap. There are several different types of ice packs.

- Homemade slush is an excellent thing to use, because it can be easily molded to the body part. Mix 4 cups of water with 1 cup of rubbing alcohol in a closeable plastic freezer bag. Place the mixture in the freezer. You can refreeze the bag and use it again.

- Frozen vegetables (peas/corn) in a bag – just as you buy them at the grocery store – mold reasonably well to the body part. Because it's not safe to eat vegetables that have been thawed and refrozen, mark the vegetable bag so you don't eat them, and you can use them again.

- Gel packs are easy to use, but they can lose their cooling effect rapidly. Follow the directions on the pack for storage and use.

Gentle self-massage. Try lightly massaging stiff or sore areas before exercise. Self-massage stimulates the skin, underlying tissues, and muscles by means of applied pressure and stretching. Slow, circular movements or light kneading motions work well for many people. Don't massage one spot for more than 10 to 15 seconds. Never massage a joint that is inflamed (hot, red, and swollen).

Use the 2-Hour Pain Rule as a guideline. If you have more pain two hours after you finish walking than before you started, then you've overdone it. Cut back on your physical activity until you find a level that does not cause more pain two hours after you finish than you had before you started. This 2-Hour Pain Rule makes sense for everyone, and you'll be reminded of it many times throughout this book. You can probably expect a little short-lived discomfort with moderate exercise, particularly if you haven't exercised in awhile. It won't damage you, and putting up with it produces good health benefits. However, if you have greatly increased, lasting, or severe pain in your hips or knees when you walk, stop and talk to your health care practitioner about it.

Use medicines for pain relief, according to your health care practitioner's advice. If you take medicines for pain relief, plan your walk for when the medicine has its greatest effect – that is, wait until the medicine has had time enough to get into your system before you start. Be sure to check with your health care practitioner before taking anything – even over-the-counter drugs – to be certain that the medicine or dosage is appropriate for you. If you get an upset stomach that doesn't go away, call your health care practitioner. There are two principal types of over-the-counter medicines for pain. Both have advantages and disadvantages

- Acetaminophen (*Tylenol*) often helps relieve minor pain or discomfort, but it does not reduce inflammation. Many people find that it doesn't upset their stomach in the way that NSAIDs can, but relatively low doses can cause liver and other problems. Something to be aware of is that it is often one of several drugs in over-the-counter cold medicines, so it can be easy to take too much if you don't read the labels carefully.

- NSAIDs (nonsteroidal anti-inflammatory drugs) such as aspirin (*Bayer*), ibuprofen (*Advil* or *Motrin*), and naproxen sodium (*Aleve*) reduce both pain and inflammation, but some people get upset stomachs and even ulcers from taking them.

Focus on something else other than your pain. To take your mind off minor discomfort when walking, think of a person's name, an animal species, an occupation, a movie title, or other items in a category for every letter of the alphabet. If you get stuck on one letter (such as X), go on to the next one. Think of a favorite song you haven't sung for a while and try to remember the lyrics. Try naming all the teams in the National Football League or the Atlantic Coast Conference or whatever you like. Plan walks with a friend

2-Hour Pain Rule

If you have more pain two hours after you finish walking than before you started, you've overdone it.

Cut back on your physical activity until you find a level that does not cause more pain.

so that you can carry on a distracting conversation. There are lots of variations of distraction, once you have the idea. However, do not distract yourself when you need to pay attention to your balance, your walking technique, or your surroundings.

Change your self-talk. All of us talk to ourselves, at least in our head, if not aloud. Our self-talk can be negative, telling ourselves things like "I can't" or "If only I didn't. . . ." Research shows that negative self-talk can worsen pain, depression, and fatigue. So try to make self-talk work for you rather than against you. Here are some examples:

Negative self-talk: "I'm stuck with this pain."

Positive self-talk: "I know what to do to make the pain get better."

Negative self-talk: "It's impossible to walk when I'm sore and tired."

Positive self-talk: "I hurt, but exercise will strengthen my body and make my joints feel better."

Reinterpret your sensations. Think specifically about your physical sensations, but try to interpret them differently. For example, analyze the precise physical sensations of "pain" or "hurt" and describe them – is the pain hot, sharp, or aching? Some other sensation?

Relabel your symptoms. See if you can begin to rename your symptoms as specific kinds of temporary discomfort, not as pain. With practice, this can help you lessen the intensity of your symptoms by training your mind to change the way it thinks about your symptoms. For example, when you first start walking, relabel the stiffness or soreness you feel as a part of getting started. Remind yourself that once you get warmed up, your joints will loosen and feel better. This is hard to do in the beginning, but it will get easier for you if you practice at times other than when walking.

"What else can I do?"

Maintain an appropriate weight. If you're overweight, consider losing excess pounds. Every extra pound on your body puts several extra pounds of pressure on your hips, knees, ankles, and feet. It also stresses your back. Although it's a long-term solution, maintaining a healthy weight usually is one of the best things anyone can do to help prevent or reduce discomfort in your back, hips, and legs.

Use elastic supports or braces. Elastic supports can be purchased at drug stores or medical supply stores. These devices can be used to provide some additional support for knees or ankles when you walk. Discuss this with your physical therapist or other health care practitioner if you're not sure. For some people, braces can provide needed knee or ankle support during exercise (just like the support braces some athletes use to protect their knees or ankles during sports activities). Be sure to wear the braces if your health care practitioner suggests them.

**3-Step
Problem-Solving
Strategy**

1 Focus on the
problem that
is most on your
mind.

2 Ask yourself: "What
might be causing
this problem? "

3 Try out different
solutions.

Discuss using a walking stick or cane with your health care practitioner. These aids can help provide stability and support as you walk, especially if you have hip or knee pain. Be sure your stick or cane is the right length. The handle or grip should reach your wrist when your hand is relaxed at your side. Check for safety. Walking sticks should be sturdy and have a broad tip. Because the tips of most canes are too small, make your cane more stable by buying a wide rubber tip at any pharmacy. Also, use it correctly – a walking stick or cane should be used on the side opposite your "bad" side.

Discuss using shoe inserts or orthotics with your health care practitioner. You can add an extra layer of cushioning in your shoes by inserting insoles that you can buy at a drugstore or shoe store. Some people may need to have special orthotic inserts in their shoes. If your feet continue to hurt, discuss this option with your health care practitioner.

Solving Other Common Difficulties

In this section, we describe some common problems that people with arthritis say they experience, and we show how you can use the 3-Step Problem-Solving Strategy to address them. We've grouped these problems and concerns into categories of worries: about your health, about where you walk, about how you feel, about what people will think, and about starting and sticking with a walking and exercise program.

Many people with arthritis use the solutions we mention here, and you will probably be able to think of many more than these examples. Pick out the problems that look most like the ones you worry about, and see if the solution examples will work for you. If not, it's also a good idea to chat with people you know who have arthritis and who exercise regularly to see what has worked for them. If you're part of a *Walk With Ease* group, share ideas with your leader and others in the group. Once you've collected the solutions that are most useful to you, you can add them to your walking plan or diary. You might also want to post them on your refrigerator or bathroom mirror, where you'll be reminded of them frequently.

Worries About Your Health

Problem: "I have medical problems."

Ask yourself: Which medical condition concerns me most? Are my symptoms or health problems severe enough that I need to consult my health care practitioner before I start my walking program?

Some solutions to try: Even with medical problems, chances are that you can do appropriate exercises. Talk with your health care practitioner or fitness professional to answer your specific questions and help develop a safe, effective program. Take this book along and use it as a basis to discuss what is right for you. Remember, nearly everyone with medical problems can and should exercise.

If you have certain severe medical conditions or symptoms, you should consult your health care practitioner before starting any form of exercise.

Problem: "My doctor hasn't told me to walk for exercise."

Ask yourself: Do I need to consult my health care practitioner before I start walking? Do I need my health care practitioner's help to plan and oversee my exercise program to make sure I am safe?

Some solutions to try: Think back: Have you ever discussed walking with your health care practitioner? Often, it never comes up! During busy office visits many health care practitioners don't think to mention something as simple as walking as a way to manage arthritis and fitness. So, it's something you need to bring up. For many people with arthritis, walking probably isn't a problem at all. Try following the guidelines and see how you feel.

If you have concerns, take this book to your health care practitioner and be prepared with specific questions to ask concerning exercise guidelines for you. Be sure to refer to overall exercise guidelines in Chapter 1 and the sections on time and intensity in the 5-Step Basic Walking Pattern in Chapter 5. Chances are you'll be able to start a program. If your health care practitioner does say you shouldn't walk, discuss alternative ways in which you can make exercise part of your life.

Problem: "My doctor said I should be careful not to overdo it when I exercise."

Ask yourself: Do I understand how I might overdo it, given my arthritis and medical conditions? Do I know my limits when it comes to exercising?

Some solutions to try: Follow the guidelines in our program, and especially review Chapters 2, 3, and 5. Start with what you can do, progress very slowly and gradually, and make changes to accommodate your form of arthritis or related condition. You can also take this book to your health care practitioner and discuss what you should do that would be within safe exercise limits for you.

Problem: "I'm afraid walking will make my arthritis worse."

Ask yourself: Do I know how to walk at my own pace? Do I know how to walk safely?

Some solutions to try: A large number of research studies now prove that appropriate exercise won't make arthritis and related conditions worse and, in fact, will help decrease overall pain and make you feel better. This is true for almost all people with arthritis: You will hurt yourself by not exercising! It is likely that regular exercise like walking will help you manage your condition and feel better. If your condition is not particularly limiting, you can start on your own and follow our recommended guidelines throughout this book. Be sure to review Chapters 1, 2 and 5. If you do have limitations, talk with your health care practitioner before starting anything. Remember to listen to your body.

Worries About Where You Walk

Problem: "The weather is too bad to go for a walk."

Ask yourself: Do I know where I can walk so I'm protected from the weather? Do I know what I can do at home to keep going on my exercise program?

Walking Location Tip

If you live in a rural area where there aren't sidewalks or there's a lot of speeding traffic, invite a buddy to drive downtown or to the mall to go walking. Downtown areas are usually well-lit and have sidewalks for walking, and malls are nice options for hot or rainy days.

Some solutions to try:

- Walk under cover in large buildings. Go to the mall. Lots of people go mall-walking, especially in bad weather. Malls provide safe, well-lit areas to walk, with water fountains, rest rooms, places to sit and rest, and plenty of scenery for window shopping and people-watching. If a mall isn't convenient, how about a supermarket, a large department store, a museum, or a convention center? Is there a community center near you or a school with an indoor track? In fact, some malls and community areas already have regularly scheduled walks during early or late hours.

- Do alternative exercises at home. Focus on your strengthening and stretching exercises when the weather is too bad to go outside. Staying active doing household chores and dancing to your favorite music will help you maintain the aerobic fitness you have achieved through your walking program.

- Plan ahead for bad weather. Remember, it never rains on a treadmill. This equipment can be purchased to substitute for outdoor walking when the weather is just too bad. Senior centers and parks and recreation centers may have them available for free or at a low cost. (Note that a treadmill may not be a good choice if you have balance problems or difficulty with your hands.) To purchase your own, consult *Consumer Reports* in your library or online, or call your YMCA for recommendations.

Problem: "I don't feel safe where I walk."

Ask yourself: Do I know where I can walk that is safe from crime? Do I know how to get help if I need it? Do I know where to go so that I can get home easily if I get tired? Do I know and use places with good walking surfaces?

Some solutions to try:

- Know the safest places to walk. It's o.k. to stay close to home. You can walk a mile by going up and down the same block several times. Avoid areas where there might be a threat to your personal safety. Use community walking areas such as schools, parks, indoor tracks or recreation centers, or walk at the mall or in a large department store.

- Be sure a family member or friend knows your walking route and approximately how long you'll be gone.

- Walk with a buddy or group. There's safety in numbers.

- Know the safest times to walk. Walk during times of day when light and shadows don't cause problems with your vision. If there's little light during your walking time, wear bright, reflective clothing or reflectors, so drivers can see you. Carry a flashlight after dusk.

- You may feel unsafe if your walking surface is uneven with lots of loose stones – a poorly maintained sidewalk, walking trail, or shoulder of a road. Be sure to review the section on walking surfaces in Chapter 3 to pick an appropriate walking surface.

> On nice days we walked outside. We had a regular walk mapped out and we followed the map. On rainy days, we improvised and walked in the church basement.
>
> *– WALK WITH EASE PARTICIPANT*

Worries About How You Feel When You're Walking

Problem: "I need to use the bathroom frequently."

Ask yourself: Do I know how to manage this problem? Do I know what works for me at other times of the day and in other situations?

Some solutions to try:

• Prepare for when you can't find a bathroom.

• Empty your bladder before you start to walk. Be careful, though, to stay hydrated when you exercise, particularly in warm weather.

• Wear appropriate pads or protective undergarments, if you usually do.

• Plan walking routes in advance, and know where the bathrooms are. If necessary, stay close to home or in areas where you know you can find a bathroom when you need one. Rather than walking where there's no bathroom, like a trail, think about doing laps around or in buildings like a mall, community center, or your house, where you can quickly get to a bathroom.

Problem: "My feet hurt."

Ask yourself: Are my shoes the problem? Am I having problems with my feet? Am I using the correct walking techniques? Is my weight making it harder for me to walk?

Some solutions to try:

- Review the shoe guidelines in Chapter 3. Make sure your shoes provide good support, are fitted properly, and are the right kind of shoe for your activity.

- Shoes wear out, and insoles wear out faster. If your shoes have a lot of miles on them, but you're not ready to replace them yet, you might consider adding an extra layer of cushioning by inserting insoles that you can buy at a drugstore or shoe store. You should replace insoles every few months to maintain good cushioning. Note: Some people may need to have special orthotic inserts in their shoes. If your feet continue to hurt, discuss this option with your health care practitioner.

- Do you have bunions, corns, plantar fasciitis (pain in your heel), arch problems, or foot conditions other than arthritis that cause discomfort? If so, see your health care practitioner for a course of treatment. Many of these problems are caused or made worse by poorly fitting shoes, so check your shoes, too. Many foot problems can be treated or corrected, so don't let them keep you from walking. Also, see the suggestions in Chapter 6 about problems that you may encounter after you've walked for awhile.

- Review the recommendations about good body mechanics in Chapter 5 and the problems walkers sometimes encounter after they've been doing it awhile in Chapter 6.

- Every extra pound on your body puts three to four extra pounds of pressure on your feet, and also on your knees, hips, and back. Maintaining a healthy weight is important for your feet and joints, and regular walking can help you maintain a good weight.

Problem: "I don't like to sweat."

Ask yourself: Why do I sweat, anyway? Do I know what to do to stay comfortable when I sweat?

Some solutions to try: Sweating is your body's natural air-conditioning system. If you sweat during exercise, it's usually a good sign. It means you're exerting yourself enough to generate energy, burn calories, and make changes that benefit your health. However, you don't have to sweat a lot to get the benefits of exercise. Remember the F.I.T.T principles discussed in Chapter 3. Low-intensity activity is fine. Just do it for a little longer. For comfort, you can wear clothing that helps absorb or wick perspiration from your body, so you don't feel as uncomfortable when you sweat. Review the clothing tips in Chapter 3 for some suggestions.

Worries About What People Will Think

Problem: "I'm stiff and unsteady on my feet. I don't like to be seen staggering."

Ask yourself: Do I know what I can do for better balance when I walk? Do I know what to do so I don't fall while I'm walking?

Some solutions to try: Consider using an aid to improve balance. If you've never used a walking stick, it might be enough to provide the support you need. Ask your health care practitioner if a walking stick would be a good aid for you.

Who cares about what inconsiderate or judgmental people think? Actually, most of us do care what others think, and we can help educate thoughtless people by being good role models. For example, call attention to your efforts by wearing an Arthritis Foundation t-shirt or one with a special exercise phrase. Seeing people with arthritis who are successfully exercising despite limitations can help others think twice about their assumptions. You'll be a great example and get your exercise. If you're still concerned, walk with a group or in an area where you are comfortable.

Problem: "I think I look ridiculous in exercise clothing."

Ask yourself: Do I need to wear exercise clothing? Do I know what I can wear that I like and that feels comfortable?

Some solutions to try: All you really need are good shoes and socks and the right amount of layers for the weather. You don't need to wear any other specific clothing – just what's comfortable for you. Some specialized exercise clothing is made of fabric that provides good support and keeps you warm, or cool, or dry, but it isn't essential that you wear it. See Chapter 3 for more ideas about what to wear.

Problem: "I'm too old or out of shape to exercise."

Ask yourself: Do I know other people my age who are exercising? Do I know where I can find information about how exercise can help people of my age? Do I know other people who are out of shape who are starting to exercise? Do

I know where I can find information about how exercise can help people who are as out of shape as I am?

Some solutions to try: It's never too late to start exercising! It doesn't matter how old or out of shape you are now – your body will receive the same benefits from walking that younger or more active people receive. Even if you have never been active before, your health will benefit as soon as you start exercising. Almost all the things that get worse with age get better with exercise, so while it's good to exercise when you're younger, it is essential to exercise as you get older. You may need to go a little slower than you might have when you were younger, but that's ok. Go at whatever speed and comfort level you need. The important thing is to get going.

Worries About Starting and Sticking With an Exercise Program

Problem: "I don't have time."

Ask yourself: Have I thought about how much time I really do need for exercise? Have I thought about flexibility in my schedule? Do I know how to combine my walks with some other activity? Have I thought about activities I could give up so I could spend more time improving my health?

Some solutions to try: Actually, few of us have the time to exercise. We have to make the time. If you work for eight to nine hours a day and sleep for another eight or nine, that leaves six to eight hours every day for other activities. Including weekends, you have 60 to 72 hours each week, but you need just two hours of that time for a great investment for your health – a small investment of time when you consider your whole week.

- Think about your schedule over a typical week and identify those times when you usually have some flexibility. Remember that you can benefit from taking three 10-minute walks, rather than having to find 30 minutes in a day. Do an experiment: See how far you can walk in 10 minutes. It may be around the block, 20 times around your living room, three times around the building where you work, or up and down all the aisles at the supermarket. You can clear your head by taking a quick walk, at home or at work.

- Combine your walk with another activity. Have a "walking meeting" with a friend or business colleague. Catch up on the news with friends or neighbors while you walk. Encourage family or friends to join you in a group walk or pace around the kitchen while you talk on the phone. If you can use a treadmill comfortably, put one in front of the TV and walk while you watch. If you have a dog, count the time you spend on walks.

- Look for activities you do now that you might be willing to give up or spend less time doing. Maybe you can give up something you don't even like!

> My *Walk With Ease* buddy and I meet at the mall, and we always walk together. Havin a buddy to walk with is a great incentive. You don't want to disappoint them.
>
> – *WALK WITH EASE PARTICIPANT*

Problem: "Other responsibilities get in the way and exercise is just not a high priority for me now."

Ask yourself: What are my responsibilities to my health? What can I do to make walking an important part of my schedule? Can I commit to making walking or other exercise a higher priority for me?

Some solutions to try: You probably have many obligations in your life – family, spouse, work, volunteer work, house work, and religious or civic activities – but if you don't stay healthy, you won't be able to meet them. A key component of staying healthy when you have arthritis is to get regular exercise. Exercising regularly will give you the energy you need to complete all the tasks on your to-do list. Exercise will reduce your pain and stiffness, help you sleep better, and boost your energy level. Having more energy can help you feel like there are more hours in your day.

- Let people know what you want and need, and get their support in helping you maintain your health. Make walking times a high priority. One good way is to make appointments with yourself by writing your walking times in your daily calendar. Keeping these appointments is just as important as keeping business meetings, doctors' appointments, or social obligations. When you tell people you can't do something because you have another appointment, most people will accept that reason.

- Many people find that scheduling walks for the same time on every exercise day helps them make walking a routine part of their schedule. Figure out a time that works best for you, whether it's early in the morning, during your lunch break, after work, or later in the evening. Put your scheduled walk on your to-do list or calendar.

- Think of walking time as a special time when you're focused on taking care of yourself. Even for just a few minutes a day, you're actively improving your health, relieving stress, and taking care of your body. Use this time to think about creative goals for yourself. Some forms of spiritual practice use "walking meditation," and that's another possible use of your walking time.

Problem: "I'm too tired."

Ask yourself: What's making me feel tired? Could it be lack of sleep, poor nutrition, too much physical exertion, side effects of certain medicines, or some other physical factor? Could it be stress, depression, or some other emotional factor? Could some combination of these physical and emotional factors be contributing to my fatigue?

Some solutions to try:

- If lack of sleep is the reason you're tired, try to go to bed earlier or get up later.

- Talk to your health care provider about your diet (and plan how to lose weight safely, if that's an issue).

- Reduce the intensity or time you spend walking, and then plan to increase it gradually.

- Ask your health care provider about your medicines.

- Lack of exercise itself can be a cause of fatigue, so you may feel less tired because you have started walking. Try just a little – one or two minutes, five minutes. If you're still too tired, stop, but you may be surprised that you have the energy to continue.

- Although it is often helpful to identify the causes of stress or depression and address them, you may find that walking makes you feel better.

- Getting help correcting underlying problems will help you feel better and have much more energy. Regular exercise really can make you more energetic. Besides making you stronger, exercise stimulates your body to pump out endorphins (the feel-good hormones) and reduces stress, both of which make you feel better and more "up and at 'em." Think of what you're not getting when you're not walking regularly.

- If you're concerned about getting too tired before you get home, consider buying a walking stick with a collapsing seat so you can rest whenever you need to. Walk in places where there are chairs or benches set a short distance apart. Remember that a walking stick not only helps with balance and joint comfort, it also is a handy defense against dogs or other aggressors. In fact, many people both with and without arthritis regularly walk with sticks for that very purpose. Check with your health care practitioner about how to select an appropriate stick or cane and use it properly.

Ok, if you really are fatigued, rest for a while. Then walk!

Problem: "I just don't feel like it."

Ask yourself: Why don't I feel like walking? Am I bored when I walk? Am I discouraged about my progress? Have I been feeling this way just today only or most of the time?

Some solutions to try: It may surprise you that even longtime, avid exercisers often don't feel like exercising either. They usually go ahead and do it, though, because they know they will feel good afterward.

- Focus on long-term achievements. Picture in your mind what you really want for yourself out of exercise. More energy? Less joint pain? Fitter body? Stronger bones? Focus on that vision, rather than on the thought that you don't feel like exercising right now.

- Discover ways to keep yourself interested. Bring a friend with you, in person or on the cell phone, and chat while you walk. Listen to music or an audiobook or the radio. However, be careful of your safety. Be sure you can also hear traffic or other outside noises and that you can pay enough attention to avoid falls or other injuries.

- Set different goals for yourself. Focus one day on improving your time, another day on alternating speeds, another day on stopping to smell the flowers, or whatever else you might enjoy.

- Mix it up! Experiment with different routes. Walk with different friends on various days of the week.

- Use your walking diary and your self-tests to help you identify progress. Even little changes can be helpful over the long term.

- Pat yourself on the back each time you go for a walk and don't forget you deserve a reward.

- Get support to carry you over the times when your motivation fails: an exercise partner, a walking group, a "cheerleader" among your family members.

- Consider getting a dog. Having to take an animal for a walk ensures that you walk, too. Studies show that dog owners have lower stress levels and live longer. Be sure to choose an animal that is appropriate in size and energy level for your own ability. Talk to a veterinarian or animal trainer for recommendations.

- If you've given walking a good try and still have trouble sticking with it, try out other types of exercises – a low-impact aerobics class, tai chi, swimming, or bicycling, for example. Talk to people you know and find out what they like to do. Maybe they're looking for company. Keep trying until you find something you think is enjoyable.

Problem: "I had to miss a few times, and it's hard to get started again."

Ask yourself: Has there been one reason for consistently missing my walks, or several different reasons? Do I know how to get back on track with my exercise routine?

Some solutions to try: Know that lapses don't have to be permanent. Even people who are dedicated to exercise have occasional times when they can't do it. If you miss doing your walks for a short time, make a firm decision to get right back on the exercise track. When people work to develop new habits (or stop doing old ones), there are predictable times when they are likely to have lapses. Realize these are coming, and plan how you will get through times when it's hard to get going by doing some of the other strategies mentioned in this section and in Chapter 6. Missing a few times is OK Just get right back with your program as soon as you can.

Remember

- Hurt does not equal harm. Use pain-management strategies to minimize hurt as much as possible. Try walking more slowly, make sure you're wearing supportive shoes, and be sure you only walk on level surfaces.

- The many benefits of exercise can be yours! By taking necessary precautions or making changes to fit your special needs, you can walk for better health and well-being.

- Your walking diary and your walking contract are helpful tools for staying focused, keeping track of what's working for you, and tracking your progress in overcoming barriers.

Self-check

TEST YOUR KNOWLEDGE
Circle either "yes" or "no" for each of the following statements:

Yes	No	I can name three physical techniques to manage my pain.
Yes	No	I can name three mental techniques to manage my pain.
Yes	No	I know how to use these techniques during my walking program.
Yes	No	I can name five ways to overcome common barriers and difficulties.

RATE YOUR CONFIDENCE LEVEL
On a scale of 0 to 10 with "0" being not confident at all and "10" being totally confident, circle the number that represents how confident you are about these statements.

I feel confident that I can manage my pain and discomfort when I'm doing my walking program.

0   1   2   3   4   5   6   7   8   9   10
Not confident at all   Totally confident

I feel confident that I have an effective plan or strategies in place to get past setbacks and obstacles to my walking plan.

0   1   2   3   4   5   6   7   8   9   10
Not confident at all   Totally confident

NEXT STEPS
Could you answer yes to the statements above? Is your confidence level 7 or more? If so, congratulations! You're ready to move on.

Each of the statements refers to a section of this chapter. If you answered no to any of them, you may wish to go back and review that section. If your confidence is low, review the sections you're not sure about. You can also share questions or concerns with your friends who have arthritis and walk or with your health care practitioner. If you're in a *Walk With Ease* group program, we recommend that you share your questions or concerns with your group leader and fellow participants.

Chapter 5

Walking With Ease!

If you've read the first four chapters of this book, you've learned about the basics about arthritis and exercising, the principles of FITT exercise, anticipating and handling problems associated with a walking program, and using motivational strategies for setting a realistic and personalized walking plan. We now turn to some practical steps for building on and maintaining your walking program, including lots of good suggestions from exercise experts for ensuring comfort, safety and success.

In this chapter, you can learn about:
- The 5-Step Basic Walking Pattern

- The Walking Progression Chart

- More tips for walking comfortably and safely

- Good body mechanics

- Strengthening and flexibility exercises

- Monitoring your exercise intensity

- Measuring your fitness level

You can also do these activities:
- Do a self-check to review your progress

- Keep your walking diary

- Review your walking plan

Implementing the 5-Step Basic Walking Pattern

As you start to implement your plan, here's some basic information to help you get off on the right foot (so to speak). Whenever you go walking for a minimum of 10 minutes, regardless of your ability or speed, follow the steps in the 5-Step Basic Walking Pattern:

5-Step Basic Walking Pattern

1 Warm up.

2 Gently stretch.

3 Walk.

4 Cool down.

5 Gently stretch again.

- Warm up by walking at a slow pace.

- Gently stretch.

- Walk.

- Cool down (allow heart rate to recover or return to a more resting level).

- Gently stretch again.

What should you do if you're accumulating 30 minutes in 10- or 15-minute walks several times a day? Be sure to warm up and cool down each time, and do the stretches at least once as day, if you can't do them each time.

Step 1: Warm up (3 to 5 minutes)

Warming up is very important before active exercise. It prepares you physically by warming up muscles and preparing you for exercise, elevating your temperature and increasing your blood flow. Warming up also prepares you mentally by helping you focus and get energized for the moderate walk to come. To warm up, all you need to do is walk at a slow pace for about three to five minutes or you may march in place. See Appendix B.

Step 2: Gently stretch
(4 to 5 minutes)

Doing leg and body stretches will help prevent shin pain, sore muscles, and other injuries, especially as you go for longer walks. We recommend four stretches before each walk: calf muscles, hamstrings, hip flexors and quadriceps, and iliotibial bands (ITBs). Be sure to do each stretch with both your right and left sides. Hold each stretch for 30 seconds on each side and do not bounce. Appendix B has pictures and directions for these stretches, some additional ones you may wish to try, as well as strengthening exercises.

Step 3: Walk
(5 to 30 minutes or more)

This is the "cardiovascular" part of your walk. Follow these guidelines:

Pick up the pace. Gradually pick up your pace until you're walking at a moderate pace. Walk as if you have somewhere to go!

Increase your time. To gradually increase your time, use the suggested walking progression chart in this chapter as a guideline. Each week add 5 minutes to your walking time. If you're a beginner, start by walking a total of 10 minutes, a three-to-five minute faster segment surrounded by your warm-up and cool-down strolls. If you already can walk for longer than 10 minutes at a time, enter the chart at your current level of walking time and go from there.

Monitor for intensity. Use the talk test described later in this chapter to monitor yourself: You should still be able to carry on a conversation even when walking at a faster pace. If you can't talk without a lot of huffing and puffing or other discomfort, your pace is too fast. Slow down to a more comfortable level.

Check your perceived exertion and/or heart rate. As you become more fit (able to walk for longer times or at a faster pace or intensity), monitor yourself at least occasionally by using the perceived exertion scale or heart rate scale, described later in the chapter. These scales help you measure how much your body is working as you exercise. Be sure to keep your heart rate within the moderate intensity level.

- Your numbers should remain in the moderate ranges – from 4 to 7 on the perceived exertion scale.

- If you have osteoarthritis, stay within the 50- to 70-percent range for your age level on the heart rate scale.

- If you have rheumatoid arthritis, try to stay within the 60- to 85-percent range for your age level on the heart rate scale.

Pay attention to your body mechanics. Body mechanics means good posture and efficient body movements. Use good body mechanics when walking. These are noted in the next section. Try to observe all techniques to help ensure safety and prevent discomfort.

Watch out for common walking errors. Avoid common walking "errors" such as overstriding (taking steps that are too long for comfort) or leaning. These also are identified in a later section in this chapter. Be sure to follow suggestions to eliminate or correct potential problems.

Step 4: Cool down (3 to 5 minutes)

At the end of your walk, slow your pace to a stroll until your heart rate has returned to your pre-walk level. Please don't skip this step, no matter how hurried you might be. A gradual cool down allows your body to "downshift" from high gear to a lower gear and finally back to the low gear of everyday movement. Cooling down lets your heart rate lower gradually and prevents your blood from pooling in your legs, which can cause light headedness, dizziness, or even fainting.

To cool down, gradually slow your walking pace to a stroll during the last 3 to 5 minutes of your walk. You should be at no more than a fairly light intensity level. (If you measure your intensity, this level would be 3 or less on the perceived exertion scale, or 10 to 14 beats on the 10-second heart rate scale.)

Step 5: Gently stretch again (7 to 9 minutes)

This is the most neglected part of a good walking program. Stretching after exercise helps you prevent soreness, increase flexibility, and maintain range of motion.

Repeat the same stretches you did during your warm up, but hold each stretch for 45 seconds to 1 minute. Do not bounce, and remember to breathe! (See Appendix B for exercise directions and pictures.)

Ideally, go through the 5-Step Basic Walking Pattern each time you walk, even if you walk in 10-minute sessions several times during the day. When your time is limited, stretch before and after walking at least one time each day you walk – before your first walk of the day might make the most sense.

Suggested Walking Progression Chart

When you can walk for a total of 10 minutes at a time (including warm up and cool down), follow this suggested walking progression chart to build your fitness program gradually. If you already can walk for longer than 10 minutes at a time, enter the chart at your current level and progress accordingly.

Week	Duration	Times/week
1	10 minutes	3–5
2	15 minutes	3–5
3	20 minutes	3–5
4	25 minutes	3–5
5	30 minutes	3–5
6	35 to 40 minutes	3–5

Always warm up and cool down by walking slowly.

Remember, this progression is a suggested goal. You may not be able to walk this long right away or progress as quickly as outlined. Or you may "top out" and be unable to add walking time beyond a certain point. That's ok. It is important to start at your current level, build up gradually, and slowly increase your time to your ability in order to increase your stamina and muscle strength.

More Tips for Walking Comfortably and Safely

Your walking program will be successful when you can walk comfortably and safely. In Chapter 4, we provided tips on what to do when exercise hurts. Some muscle soreness often develops a day or two after you exercise, particularly if you're just beginning your program. Take warm baths, stretch gently, and continue to walk. Here are more tips for handling symptoms, physical needs, or other problems:

Watch for serious danger signs. If you feel any of the following symptoms, stop immediately. These are danger signs. If they persist, get medical help or call 911.

- severe pain

- pressure, tightness, or pain in your chest

- nausea

- difficulty with breathing

- dizziness

- severe trembling

- light-headedness.

Watch your exertion level. If you have any of the following symptoms, slow down immediately. These are signs you're overexerting yourself. Cut back on your walking intensity or time the next time you exercise.

- cramps or stitches in your side

- very red face

- sudden paling or blanching

- profuse sweating

- facial expression signifying distress

- extreme tiredness

- fatigue or joint pain that lasts two hours after exercising (and is greater than you had before you started).

Know your body's normal reactions to moderate exercise. These reactions to moderate exercise are normal, so it's OK to continue.

- increased breathing

- increased heart rate

- increased perspiration

- muscle soreness.

Empty your bladder before you begin. Always empty your bladder before exercising. Note: if you frequently have to go to the bathroom or experience the common dilemma of "leaking," see suggestions in Chapter 4.

Drink plenty of fluids. Most people should drink plenty of fluids after each workout, whether you feel thirsty or not. Water is essential to satisfy your body's need for fluid, especially when you perspire. If it's very hot or you know you're going to be walking for a long time, you might want to take along a water bottle in a fanny pack or backpack. Be especially aware of drinking enough water when you walk in humid weather, since you're less conscious of fluid loss.

Menstruation. It is perfectly safe to exercise when you're menstruating. In fact, many women find that exercise helps reduce cramps or other uncomfortable menstrual symptoms.

Plan for contingencies. If you're unable to walk during one of your planned times because of weather or emergencies, that's OK, but decide immediately when you will schedule your next session.

Pace yourself. Remember that symptoms of arthritis come and go. Exercise that seems easy one day may seem too hard the next. When this happens, cut back temporarily and then return to your regular program when you can.

Good Body Mechanics

Good body mechanics are efficient movements that produce the least stress on your body and reduce the likelihood of injuries or problems. From your head to your toes, the following are some tips to keep your body moving well.

Head. Keep your head up. Don't jut your head forward or lead with your chin.

Shoulders. Periodically think about your shoulders to be sure they are relaxed and down (not hunched). If you're hunching, lift your rib cage up and do a few backward shoulder circles to relax your shoulders.

Lungs. Breathe deeply from your lungs and diaphragm. Avoid shallow breathing with only your upper lungs.

Stomach. Tighten your stomach muscles lightly to maintain good back support.

Arms. Swing your arms naturally and easily at your sides, with your arms moving opposite to your legs (i.e., your right arm swings forward as you step with your left leg, then your left arm swings forward as you step with your right leg).

Hands. Don't clench your fists. Just hold your hands naturally. If you have a tendency to clench, imagine you have fragile raw eggs in your hands as you swing your arms naturally.

Legs. Be careful not to take strides that are too long, which wastes energy and increases impact. Especially avoid the natural tendency to take longer strides as you become more fit, or when it's a beautiful day and you just feel great! Take regular, natural steps that are comfortable with your tempo. If you need to reduce impact, take even shorter steps.

Strengthening and Flexibility Exercises

Remember that this book focuses on the development of a walking program and does not contain information about other kinds of strengthening and flexibility exercises you would be doing as part of your arthritis management program. Chapter 6 and Appendix C contain other exercise program suggestions. If you have ongoing, severe pain in your knees, ankles, or hips, you should talk to your health care practitioner to get specific exercise recommendations.

Monitoring Your Exercise Intensity

Monitoring intensity when you exercise is good for two reasons: (1) it lets you know if you're working hard enough or too hard, so that you exercise at a safe and effective level, and (2) it helps provide you with a measuring stick to gauge your progress over time.

There are several good and easy ways to measure your exercise intensity level. Here are three techniques with an explanation of how to use each of them. When appropriate, we also tell you about any special considerations that might make the test less effective for you.

Monitoring Technique 1: The Talk Test

How to use it: This is a quick, informal way to make sure you're not overdoing it. Simply talk out loud to another person or yourself, sing or recite the verse of a poem or song lyric while you walk. Low- or moderate-intensity exertion allows you to speak comfortably, without huffing and puffing or being out of breath. If you can't carry on a conversation or sing because you're short of breath or breathing too heavily, you're working too hard. Slow down!

Over time, you'll probably find that you can exert yourself harder or for longer durations and still be able to talk comfortably. That's an easy way to measure your progress.

Special considerations: This method is not effective if you have asthma or another problem related to breathing. If so, you should use the perceived exertion or heart rate scales described here.

Monitoring Technique 2: The Perceived Exertion Scale

How to use it: The perceived exertion scale allows you to be more specific than the talk test in determining the intensity of your exercise. With perceived exertion, people score intensity based on how they feel.

To use this scale, look at the descriptions and pick one that best describes your level of exertion, and then look at the numeric rating that matches. For example, if you stated that the effort you were exerting was at the "hard" level, the corresponding number to this would be 9. If you're brand-new to walking and exercise or if you have significant limitations or are older, you should begin walking at a "very light" level (2) or at most a "fairly light" level (3) of exertion for you. That would be a slow walk or stroll. Over time, gradually increase your exertion level to walk at a "moderate/somewhat hard" level (4 to 7). Even if you are very fit, do not exercise at a level you would describe as "hard," "very hard," or "very, very hard." At those levels you risk injuring yourself.

Ideally, you should take a copy of this scale with you and check your perceived level of exertion when you're walking, but you can also measure it just before you begin your cool down.

Monitoring Technique 3: Heart Rate Scale

How to use it: For most people, monitoring your intensity by taking your pulse and using the heart rate scale is the most accurate way to measure your cardiac intensity. By finding out what your target heart rate is you ensure that you're working at

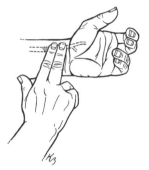

a safe and effective level for you. Moderate cardiac intensity – the kind of walking that is recommended for health and fitness – should raise your heart rate into a range between 60 and 75 percent of your maximum heart rate. This range is called your target heart rate and is the recommended level for walking for most people with arthritis.

Perceived Exertion Scale

Verbal description of your exertion	Numeric rating of your exertion
Nothing at all (such as lying down)	0
Very, very light (practically nothing)	1
Very light	2
Fairly light	3
Moderate (still light but starting to work a little more)	4
Moderate (still comfortable but harder)	5
Moderate (getting to be somewhat hard)	6
Somewhat hard	7
Hard	8
Very hard	9
Very, very hard (couldn't do for more than a few seconds)	10

Be aware that maximum heart rate declines with age, so your safe target heart rate gets lower as you get older. You can use the target heart rate scale and the steps outlined here to find your target heart rate.

How to take your pulse: You should measure your heart rate a few minutes into your exercise program to determine how much you're exerting yourself. To use the heart rate scale to monitor walking, you need to know how to take your pulse for 10 seconds. You'll need a clock or watch with a second hand.

Here are the steps for a 10-second heart rate count:

- Take your pulse by placing the pads of your index and middle fingers on your wrist below the base of your thumb. Do not use your thumb to take your pulse because it has its own pulse and will get in the way of counting of your actual pulse. You should be able to feel your blood pumping and the "thump" of your heart beating.

- Get your clock or watch ready, and for 10 seconds count how many beats you feel. Begin your count with zero for the first beat you feel.

- Multiply your number of heartbeats by 6 to find out how many times your heart is beating in one minute. Example: if you counted 13 heartbeats, multiply 13 by 6, which equals 78. So your heart rate would be 78.

- Your number should fall within the 60 percent to 75 percent range of numbers for your age level on the Target Heart Rate Scale. If your number is too high, you're exercising too intensely. Slow down. If your number is too low, and you feel ok, you can work harder.

Target Heart Rate Scale

Age	Max Heart Rate	One Minute Count		10-Second Count	
		60% of max	75% of max	60% of max	75% of max
20–24	200	120	150	20	25
25–29	195	117	146	19	24
30–34	190	114	142	19	24
35–39	185	111	139	18	23
40–44	180	108	135	18	22
45–49	175	105	131	17	22
50–54	170	102	127	17	21
55–59	165	99	124	16	21
60–64	160	96	120	16	20
65–69	155	93	116	15	19
70–74	150	90	112	15	19
75+	145	87	108	14	18

Some people have trouble increasing their heart rate, even to the 60 percent level, particularly at first. Don't worry about that. As you become experienced and stronger, your heart rate will rise because you're exercising more vigorously.

Special considerations: If you're pregnant or taking medicines that affect your heart rate, the target heart rate scale will not be accurate. Instead, monitor your exercise intensity by using the talk test or the rate of perceived exertion scale. Here are some types of medicines that may affect the accuracy of the scale:

• Heart medicines

• High blood pressure medicines

• Medicines for depression, anxiety, or other mood disorders

• Cold medicines

• Diet medicines

• Medicines to help your breathing (for asthma, COPD, etc.)

Measuring Your Fitness Level

The main reason for measuring your fitness level is that it gives you a good gauge of your progress, especially if you do this at the beginning and ending points of your walking contract, as outlined in Chapter 3. Measuring your fitness level is easy. There are three good methods.

1. Measure how far you can walk during a set period of time.

2. Walk a specific distance and see how long it takes.

3. Measure your heart rate after you've been walking for a certain amount of time.

Here's the equipment you'll need:

- A watch with a second hand or a stopwatch to take your pulse count and to measure time if you're walking a specific distance

- A pedometer, car odometer, or another way to measure distance if you're walking for a designated amount of time

- A pencil and paper to record time and/or pulse rate

- Comfortable walking shoes and clothing

Measuring may sound complicated, but it really isn't. Follow these steps.

1. Choose which method you're going to use. Pick either a length of time that you can walk without stopping – for example, 10 minutes – or, set a distance that you can complete, no matter how long it would take – for example, around the block 10 times, or up to the corner and back.

2. Find a smooth, level surface where you can measure your distance fairly accurately, such as a track, neighborhood streets, or your local shopping mall. Try to avoid lots of stoplights and heavy traffic areas. If you can't avoid these, that's OK. Just continue to march lightly in place while you wait for any delays.

3. Warm up and stretch, using the same warm up that you do before each walking session (see Appendix B).

4. Write down the time you start and the place you're starting. It's important that you try not to stop at any time during the test. If you're getting tired, slow down as much as you need to, even down to a very slow walk, but keep walking until you have completed your entire time or distance. If you do need to stop, that's fine – you'll now have a better idea of what is doable for you. Do your test on another day, and choose a better distance or time for you.

5. If you've set a predetermined walking time, note where you are – for example, "in front of the yellow house or at the corner of First and Elm." Keep moving slowly for a few minutes and then stretch to cool down. Then, measure the distance you traveled during that time, either by using a pedometer, your car odometer, or counting the number of times you circled the track or mall. Note the distance on your contract or in your diary.

6. If you're walking for a predetermined distance, note the time that you reached your stopping point. Keep moving slowly for a few minutes and then stretch to cool down. Record the time it took to walk your distance in minutes and seconds.

7. If you choose to use the heart rate scale, take your pulse for ten seconds before you start your cool down. Multiply by 6 or use the conversion chart on the scale above to determine your beats per minute. Then record your one-minute pulse rate.

We suggest you measure your fitness level several times during the six-week program – in weeks 2, 4, and 6. If you don't see improvements between your first and second measurement, it's OK. It may take some time, and the important thing is that you're being active.

That's it! At regular times during your plan – or at least at the end of the time you specified in your contract – take the fitness test to track your progress. You probably will see that you can walk for a longer distance during your designated time. On the other hand, you may find you're able to complete the same distance in a shorter time. Record the time it took to walk your distance in minutes and seconds. Either way, that's a sign of improvement in your fitness level. If you don't see any change, that's OK. You may be at a level that is just right for you, and which you can continue comfortably.

Remember

- When it comes to exercise, keep telling yourself, "I can do this!" It's only 30 minutes of walking a day, at least five days a week to make your joints, bones, muscles and heart fitter and healthier. That's less than two hours out of the entire 168 hours in a week. For the remaining hours in the week, you'll feel better, experience less pain, have more energy, be stronger, and have a brighter emotional outlook as a result of the time you've spent walking.

- Your walking diary is an important tool for tracking your exercise intensity and fitness.

Self-check

Test Your Knowledge
Circle either "yes" or "no" for each of the following statements:

Yes	No	I understand the importance of all five steps of the walking pattern.
Yes	No	I understand good walking principles and body mechanics.
Yes	No	I know how to measure my walking intensity.
Yes	No	I know how to measure my fitness level.
Yes	No	I understand the importance of recognizing exercise limitations and safety considerations.

RATE YOUR CONFIDENCE LEVEL

On a scale of 0 to 10 with "0" being not confident at all and "10" being totally confident, circle the number that represents how confident you are about these statements.

I feel confident that I can follow the 5-Step Basic Walking Pattern on my own.

0   1   2   3   4   5   6   7   8   9   10
Not confident at all   Totally confident

I feel confident that I can maintain good body mechanics when I walk.

0   1   2   3   4   5   6   7   8   9   10
Not confident at all   Totally confident

I feel confident that I can monitor my walking intensity.

0   1   2   3   4   5   6   7   8   9   10
Not confident at all   Totally confident

I feel confident that I can measure my fitness level.

0   1   2   3   4   5   6   7   8   9   10
Not confident at all   Totally confident

NEXT STEPS

Could you answer yes to the statements? Is your confidence level 7 or more? If so, congratulations! You're ready to move on.

Each of the statements refers to a section of this chapter. If you answered no to any of them, you may wish to go back and review that section. If your confidence is low, review the sections you're not sure about. You can also share questions or concerns with your friends who have arthritis and walk or with your health care practitioner. If you're in a *Walk With Ease* group program, we recommend that you share your questions or concerns with your group leader and fellow participants.

Chapter 6

Resources to Keep You Walking and Active

The motivation to stick with a walking program is not some mysterious thing that some people have and others do not. The real way to achieve success is to set goals and rewards, find ways to overcome problems, and build supports that will keep you motivated. Here are several strategies that may help:

- Develop and maintain support among your family and friends or participate in exercise programs.

- Avoid injuries by following exercise guidelines and watching out for physical problems.

- Learn about other physical activity programs that can provide support.

- Learn how to get yourself started again, if you stop for awhile.

- Make a plan for walking, use it, and update it regularly.

This final chapter provides information on each of these strategies. Together, these strategies can help you keep walking for a lifetime after you complete the six weeks of the *Walk With Ease* program.

In this chapter, you can learn about:
- Developing and maintaining support

- Watching out for physical problems

- Getting involved in other arthritis and activity programs

- Making a plan for your future

- What to do if you stop and need to get going again

You can also do these activities:
- Do your Ending Point Self-test

- Do a self-check to review your progress

- Make a plan for continuing to walk and exercise

- Keep on walking!

Developing and Maintaining Support

You have a greater chance of keeping up your walking plan successfully if your family, friends, and co-workers support your efforts. You can generate your own cheering squad by planning to include specific individuals.

Your spouse or partner is probably one of the most important people in your life. He or she can have a major impact on helping you maintain motivation. Ask your partner to join you on some of your walks. Discuss daily events, family issues, or the news. Both of you will reap the benefits of walking, and the time you spend together may have other benefits as well.

Family members can help. Do you have children or grandchildren? Take them for a walk, to the park or the zoo, or on some other outing that requires walking. Besides getting your own walk, you'll be serving as a good example that physical activity is fun and important. And remember, adult children like these things, too.

Friends and co-workers can become exercise buddies. Arrange for a morning walk with a friend. It's not as easy to roll over and go back to sleep if you know your exercise partner is waiting. Meet a co-worker at lunchtime and walk together to a cafeteria or restaurant nearby.

Exercise role models. No, these aren't star athletes or famous movie stars, but real people you admire for their walking and exercise habits. Maybe you have a friend who has severe arthritis but who walks regularly. If you walk with a group, maybe one of the members is particularly motivated. Talk to these people about how and why they keep to their walking program. If they can do it, so can you.

Walking group. If you don't belong to one already, think about joining a *Walk With Ease* group. If there isn't one in your area, think about starting one. Contact your local office of the Arthritis Foundation for more information.

Watching Out for Physical Problems

Everyone, regardless of age, level of ability, or experience, should follow recommended guidelines for safety and comfort when exercising. Many safety recommendations for starting your walking program have already been covered in this book. The chart on the next page shows a few problems you may encounter as you build up your minutes or distance. Also, here are a few things people sometimes do when they walk that also can cause problems;

Overstriding. If your hair or hat bounces up and down when you walk, it's a good indication you're overstriding. Sometimes when you feel great and you're enjoying yourself, you may have a natural tendency to do this, but remember, it increases impact and adds stress to your hips, knees, and feet. Try to glide along the ground and take shorter, more natural steps.

Elbow whipping. A good arm swing comes naturally from the shoulder, not up and down from the elbow. While it's fine to keep your elbows in a comfortable, natural bend, avoid "whipping" the forearms up and down from a bent elbow. Avoid a "rocking the baby" motion, if you can.

My *Walk With Ease* buddy encouraged me to go because I was having a little trouble with my back. She thought that walking would be good for it, and it really turned out to be true. She encouraged me to walk. After we finished the program, we also just kept walking outside, which we continue to do today. She's been a great inspiration.

– WALK WITH EASE PARTICIPANT

Common Problems and What To Do

Problem	Why it happens	What to do
Sore shins (shin splints)	Shoes that are too big or that provide poor support	Be sure your shoes fit properly If you find yourself "gripping" your shoes with your toes, it's a sign that your shoes may be too big. (See Chapter 3.)
	Inadequate warming up and stretching	Start walking with a strolling warm-up and stretch; always cool down gradually and stretch again. Do ankle flexibility exercises and stretch your shins daily. (See Appendix B.)
	Doing too much, too fast	Increase your walking time slowly. Slow down, if necessary.
Sore knees	Walking too fast	Slow down a little and keep your stride short. To slow your speed but keep your heart rate up, try doing more work with your arms (but avoid "elbow whipping, see below).
	Walking on a surface that's too stressful	Review the section "A Note About Impact" in Chapter 3 and find a place with a better surface for your walks.
	Shoes that don't fit right	Be sure your shoes provide good support and cushioning. (See Chapter 3.)
Calf Cramps	Not enough stretching before and after walking	Warm up and stretch properly.
	Dehydration – not enough water in your system	Drink enough water while you exercise
	Circulatory problems in your legs	Walk briskly for awhile, and then walk slowly for a while. Consult your health care practitioner if they don't get better as your fitness improves.
Heel Pain	Inadequate stretching	Warm up. Stretch. (See stretches in Appendix B.)
	Poor arch support	Shoes with better support and cushioning. If it doesn't go away as your fitness improves, consult with your health care practitioner.

Waist leaning. An ache in your lower back after walking often is the result of tilting forward at the waist and letting your buttocks stick out. You will lean forward a bit when you walk, but the lean should be from your ankles. To feel the difference in position, stand with your back against a wall and then lean slightly forward while leaving your buttocks against the wall. Then stand with your back against the wall and lean slightly forward from your ankles – that's the proper forward lean.

Slumping puts pressure on your back and keeps you from breathing as deeply as you might. Review the section on good body mechanics in Chapter 5. Remember: Keep your chest up, abdominal muscles in, and shoulders relaxed and down.

I like to walk, but I don't like to walk by myself. It's nice to walk with people. I really enjoy it.

– WALK WITH EASE PARTICIPANT

Getting Involved in Other Arthritis and Activity Programs

People who become involved in one type of physical activity and find that they like it often go on to explore other kinds of activity programs that are enjoyable and offer health benefits. There are many possible sources of these programs – through local parks and recreation departments, wellness centers, and senior centers, just to name a few.

Local chapters of national organizations also sponsor programs you might want to try out. Here is a brief description of three of them, and there are more suggestions in Appendix C.

- The Arthritis Foundation offers a variety of programs through its local chapters for people at different levels of fitness. Among them is the eight-week Arthritis Foundation Exercise Program, the Arthritis Foundation

Aquatic Program (exercises in a swimming pool), and Arthritis Foundation Tai Chi Program. Through the Arthritis Self-Management Program, people learn how to manage arthritis better, communicate well with health care providers, and share experiences with others. Call 800-283-7800 or visit www.arthritis.org to find your nearest Arthritis Foundation office to learn more about these programs and where they're offered. (For more information about the Arthritis Foundation's programs, see Appendix C.)

- In addition to the Arthritis Foundation programs, the Centers for Disease Control and Prevention recommends two other programs that many participants have found to improve their fitness, increase their activity levels, and improve their outlook on life. These are EnhanceFitness (EF) (formerly Lifetime Fitness) and the Chronic Disease Self-Management Program. To find out about availability of these programs in your state, you can visit the CDC Arthritis Program Web site at www.cdc.gov/arthritis.

- AARP offers two free programs on the Internet that help you track your progress. If you participate in Get Fit on Route 66, you can log your minutes of exercise and convert them to miles on a virtual journey along America's most famous highway. If you participate in Step Up to Better Health, you use a step counter to track your progress along one of four famous American trails. Learn more about these programs at the AARP Web site, www. aarp.org/walking.

Making a Plan for Your Future

This entire book has been designed to help you develop the kind of walking program that is safe, effective, and doable. It's a program that you'll be able to keep up for a lifetime of better health.

If you've been walking for six weeks or more, this is the time for you to make an "ending point" assessment of your progress and to make a new contract for your new and continuing goals.

To help you assess your ending point, we recommend that you again fill out the Ending Point Self-test Tool that's at the end of this chapter. It's like the one you completed in Chapter 1 when you assessed your starting point. Compare your results now with your results from the beginning of the program. Do you see any improvements in your pain or fatigue? Do you see any improvements in your ability to function with arthritis? It's ok if you don't see much change yet, particularly if doing a walking program is a new activity for you. Give it some time – maybe another three weeks – and do the Ending Point Self-test again. (We've also provided a copy in Appendix A that you can photocopy and use in the future to measure improvement as you keep walking). If you do see some change, congratulations! You're on the right track. Use this information to help you decide what your new goals are and what you will do to maintain your successful walking program.

At the end of six weeks, evaluate your progress with your Ending Point Self-test, and plan your next goals!

We pointed out in Chapter 3 that people find that writing down their plans helps them to focus their thoughts, reminds them what they want to do, and provides a way to keep them on track. They also find that spelling out rewards – and making sure they get rewarded – is a very important part of sticking to their plans. Think about and make a new contract with yourself like the one you completed for the first six weeks of the program. There's a place in week 6 of your diary to review all six weeks of your program. (There is a blank Contract and Walking Diary form in Appendix A for you to use if you wish.)

To help you focus your thinking, ask these questions. You might want to make notes of your answers here or on your diary.

- What progress have I made in meeting my goals?

- What are realistic goals for the next 3 months of walking?

- What are steps I can take to meet those goals?

- What information, tips, and tools from this book will be most useful to me?

- What other information and resources will be most useful to me?

- Who can help support me to continue my walking program and how can they help me?

- What reward will I get for accomplishing my goals?

- What is my confidence level in accomplishing these goals?

"But what if I stop? How do I start again?"

People find it hard to change habits – whether to get rid of an unhealthy one like smoking or to develop a new healthy one like walking regularly. Also, you have a real life, and things happen that can keep you from doing all the things you want or intend to do. If you find that you aren't walking as regularly as you'd like – or at all – and you want to do more or get started again, here are some suggestions.

1. Be nice to yourself – no shame, no blame for not doing as much as you had hoped.

2. If you can use the problem-solving method we suggested in Chapters 1 and 4 to identify the barrier that got in your way, do it, because it may help you avoid hitting it again. Otherwise, put the past behind you – it's a new day.

3. Start slowly, particularly if it has been awhile since you've been able to walk regularly. Review your last walking diary, Ending Point Self-test, and contract, and set a new goal. However, don't start exactly where you left off. Take it a little easier than where you were before, and build back up to your old level gradually.

4. Find people or programs to support you.

5. Set small goals to begin with, and reward yourself (and get your support people to reward you) for accomplishing them.

Final Thoughts

So it's now up to you!

- When you need to, review all of the chapters for suggestions concerning good exercise techniques and safety.

- Discuss any questions you have with your health care practitioner.

- Always remember to move at your own pace. Progress slowly and gradually.

- Remember to use your walking plan and diary as tools to help you stay on track and gauge your progress.

- Be sure to use the techniques for monitoring your exercise intensity and measuring your fitness level.

- Do your best, challenge yourself if you can, but don't try to keep up with anyone else.

Remember

- Your overall program should include three basic kinds of exercise: flexibility, strengthening, and cardiovascular exercises.

- You will not cause damage to yourself with appropriate exercise.

- You can cause damage to yourself by not exercising!

- Hurt does not equal harm.

- Setbacks are normal.

- Developing a plan to succeed will improve your chances of success.

- Be sure to give yourself a congratulatory reward for your dedication and success.

- The many benefits of exercise can be yours! By taking necessary precautions or making changes to fit your special needs, you can walk for better health and well-being. Your *Walk With Ease* program is for you from now on, to help you manage your arthritis and become healthier and fit!

Self-check

TEST YOUR KNOWLEDGE
Circle either "yes" or "no" for each of the following statements:

Yes	No	I can explain the importance of having a good support system for my walking program.
Yes	No	I know how to watch out for physical problems that can occur with walking and exercise.
Yes	No	I know about some of the other types of programs available for people with arthritis that I could join.
Yes	No	I know some strategies for getting started again, if I need them.

RATE YOUR CONFIDENCE LEVEL
On a scale of 0 to 10 with "0" being not confident at all and "10" being totally confident, circle the number that represents how confident you are about these statements.

I feel confident that I can develop a support system that helps me keep going.

0	1	2	3	4	5	6	7	8	9	10
Not confident at all								Totally confident		

I feel confident that I know where to look for the Arthritis resources I need.

0	1	2	3	4	5	6	7	8	9	10
Not confident at all								Totally confident		

I feel confident I can keep up my walking program.

0	1	2	3	4	5	6	7	8	9	10
Not confident at all								Totally confident		

NEXT STEPS
Could you answer yes to the statements above? Is your confidence level 7 or more? If so, congratulations! You're ready to move on.

Each of the statements refers to a section of this chapter. If you answered no to any of them, you may wish to go back and review that section. If your confidence is low, review the sections you're not sure about. You can also share questions or concerns with your friends who have arthritis and walk or with your health care practitioner. If you're in a *Walk With Ease* group program, we recommend that you share your questions or concerns with your group leader and fellow participants.

Ending Point Self-test

Do you see any improvement from your Starting Point Self-test?

PAIN
Please circle the number that describes how much physical pain your arthritis has caused during the past week.

0	1	2	3	4	5	6	7	8	9	10

No pain   As bad as it can be

FATIGUE
Please circle the number that describes how much of a problem fatigue has been for you during the past week.

0	1	2	3	4	5	6	7	8	9	10

No problem   A major problem

PHYSICAL LIMITATIONS
The following items are about activities you might do during a typical day. Does your health now *limit* you in these activities? If so, how much? (Circle one number on each line.)

	Not at all	Yes, a little	Yes, a lot
Vigorous activities, such as running, lifting heavy objects, participating in strenuous sports	1	2	3
Moderate activities, such as moving a table, pushing a vacuum cleaner, bowling, or playing golf	1	2	3
Lifting or carrying groceries	1	2	3
Climbing *several* flights of stairs	1	2	3
Climbing *one* flight of stairs	1	2	3
Bending, kneeling, or stooping	1	2	3
Walking *more* than a mile	1	2	3
Walking *several hundred yards*	1	2	3
Walking *one hundred yards*	1	2	3
Bathing or dressing yourself	1	2	3

Add up all the circled numbers and write your total Physical Limitations score in the box:

Ending Point Self-test Scoring Instructions

PAIN
If your score was:

1–3   Pain is probably not your main concern. You may want to make pain management a lower priority for now and focus on other topics in the book.

4–7   Pain is probably an important concern for you. Many of the suggestions in this book will help you to reduce your pain. Information on pain management can be found in Chapters 4 and 6.

8–10   Pain is probably a main problem for you. Tell your health care practitioner that you're experiencing a lot of pain. Medication or a change in medication may help. Many of the suggestions in this book will help you to manage your pain. Information on pain management can be found in Chapters 4 and 6.

FATIGUE
1–3   Fatigue is probably not your main concern. You may want to make fatigue management a lower priority for now and focus on other topics in the book.

4-7   Fatigue is probably an important concern for you. Many of the suggestions in this book will help you to reduce your fatigue. Information on fatigue management can be found in Chapters 4 and 6.

8–10   Fatigue is probably a main problem for you. Tell your health care practitioner if you're experiencing a lot of fatigue. Some medications may cause fatigue. Information on fatigue management can be found in Chapters 4 and 6.

PHYSICAL LIMITATIONS
10–15   You probably don't have many physical limitations. Information in Chapter 5 and the exercises in Appendix B will give you ideas for improving your muscle flexibility, strength, and endurance.

16–22   You have some physical limitations, which can probably be improved if you increase your muscle flexibility, strength, and endurance. Chapter 5 and the exercises in Appendix B will give you ideas for improving your muscle flexibility, strength, and endurance.

23–30   You have many physical limitations. The good news is that consistent exercise will probably help you improve your physical activities. Information in Chapter 5 and the exercises in Appendix B may give you ideas for improving your muscle flexibility, strength, and endurance, but check with your health care practitioner for more suggestions.

Appendix A

Self-tests, Contracts, and Diaries

Starting Point Self-test

PAIN
Please circle the number that describes how much physical pain your arthritis has caused during the past week.

0   1   2   3   4   5   6   7   8   9   10

No pain   As bad as it can be

FATIGUE
Please circle the number that describes how much of a problem fatigue has been for you during the past week.

0   1   2   3   4   5   6   7   8   9   10

No problem   A major problem

PHYSICAL LIMITATIONS
The following items are about activities you might do during a typical day. Does your health now **limit** you in these activities? If so, how much? (Circle one number on each line.)

	Not at all	Yes, a little	Yes, a lot
Vigorous activities, such as running, lifting heavy objects, participating in strenuous sports	1	2	3
Moderate activities, such as moving a table, pushing a vacuum cleaner, bowling, or playing golf	1	2	3
Lifting or carrying groceries	1	2	3
Climbing *several* flights of stairs	1	2	3
Climbing *one* flight of stairs	1	2	3
Bending, kneeling, or stooping	1	2	3
Walking *more* than a mile	1	2	3
Walking *several hundred yards*	1	2	3
Walking *one hundred yards*	1	2	3
Bathing or dressing yourself	1	2	3

Add up all the circled numbers and write your total Physical Limitations score in the box:

Starting Point Self-test Scoring Instructions

PAIN

If your score was:

1–3   Pain is probably not your main concern. You may want to make pain management a lower priority for now and focus on other topics in the book.

4–7   Pain is probably an important concern for you. Many of the suggestions in this book will help you to reduce your pain. Information on pain management can be found in Chapters 4 and 6.

8–10   Pain is probably a main problem for you. Tell your health care practitioner that you're experiencing a lot of pain. Medication or a change in medication may help. Many of the suggestions in this book will help you to manage your pain. Information on pain management can be found in Chapters 4 and 6.

FATIGUE

1–3   Fatigue is probably not your main concern. You may want to make fatigue management a lower priority for now and focus on other topics in the book.

4-7   Fatigue is probably an important concern for you. Many of the suggestions in this book will help you to reduce your fatigue. Information on fatigue management can be found in Chapters 4 and 6.

8–10   Fatigue is probably a main problem for you. Tell your health care practitioner if you're experiencing a lot of fatigue. Some medications may cause fatigue. Information on fatigue management can be found in Chapters 4 and 6.

PHYSICAL LIMITATIONS

10–15   You probably don't have many physical limitations. Information in Chapter 5 and the exercises in Appendix B will give you ideas for improving your muscle flexibility, strength, and endurance.

16–22   You have some physical limitations, which can probably be improved if you increase your muscle flexibility, strength, and endurance. Chapter 5 and the exercises in Appendix B will give you ideas for improving your muscle flexibility, strength, and endurance.

23–30   You have many physical limitations. The good news is that consistent exercise will probably help you improve your physical activities. Information in Chapter 5 and the exercises in Appendix B may give you ideas for improving your muscle flexibility, strength, and endurance, but check with your health care practitioner for more suggestions.

Ending Point Self-test

Do you see any improvement from your Starting Point Self-test?

_____

PAIN
Please circle the number that describes how much physical pain your arthritis has caused during the past week.

0   1   2   3   4   5   6   7   8   9   10
No pain   As bad as it can be

FATIGUE
Please circle the number that describes how much of a problem fatigue has been for you during the past week.

0   1   2   3   4   5   6   7   8   9   10
No problem   A major problem

PHYSICAL LIMITATIONS
The following items are about activities you might do during a typical day. Does your health now *limit* you in these activities? If so, how much? (Circle one number on each line.)

	Not at all	Yes, a little	Yes, a lot
Vigorous activities, such as running, lifting heavy objects, participating in strenuous sports	1	2	3
Moderate activities, such as moving a table, pushing a vacuum cleaner, bowling, or playing golf	1	2	3
Lifting or carrying groceries	1	2	3
Climbing *several* flights of stairs	1	2	3
Climbing *one* flight of stairs	1	2	3
Bending, kneeling, or stooping	1	2	3
Walking *more* than a mile	1	2	3
Walking *several hundred yards*	1	2	3
Walking *one hundred yards*	1	2	3
Bathing or dressing yourself	1	2	3

Add up all the circled numbers and write your total Physical Limitations score in the box: ☐

Ending Point Self-test Scoring Instructions

PAIN
If your score was:

1–3   Pain is probably not your main concern. You may want to make pain management a lower priority for now and focus on other topics in the book.

4–7   Pain is probably an important concern for you. Many of the suggestions in this book will help you to reduce your pain. Information on pain management can be found in Chapters 4 and 6.

8–10   Pain is probably a main problem for you. Tell your health care practitioner that you're experiencing a lot of pain. Medication or a change in medication may help. Many of the suggestions in this book will help you to manage your pain. Information on pain management can be found in Chapters 4 and 6.

FATIGUE

1–3   Fatigue is probably not your main concern. You may want to make fatigue management a lower priority for now and focus on other topics in the book.

4-7   Fatigue is probably an important concern for you. Many of the suggestions in this book will help you to reduce your fatigue. Information on fatigue management can be found in Chapters 4 and 6.

8–10   Fatigue is probably a main problem for you. Tell your health care practitioner if you're experiencing a lot of fatigue. Some medications may cause fatigue. Information on fatigue management can be found in Chapters 4 and 6.

PHYSICAL LIMITATIONS

10–15   You probably don't have many physical limitations. Information in Chapter 5 and the exercises in Appendix B will give you ideas for improving your muscle flexibility, strength, and endurance.

16–22   You have some physical limitations, which can probably be improved if you increase your muscle flexibility, strength, and endurance. Chapter 5 and the exercises in Appendix B will give you ideas for improving your muscle flexibility, strength, and endurance.

23–30   You have many physical limitations. The good news is that consistent exercise will probably help you improve your physical activities. Information in Chapter 5 and the exercises in Appendix B may give you ideas for improving your muscle flexibility, strength, and endurance, but check with your health care practitioner for more suggestions.

Contract

From (date): _____ To: _____

I, _____ plan to walk

_____ days a week

for _____ minutes a day or _____ (distance),

broken into _____ sessions.

I plan to walk _____

(time of day, e.g., at lunch, after dinner).

I will spend 3 to 5 minutes warming up and

4 to 5 minutes doing warm-up stretches

and 3 to 5 minutes cooling down and

7 to 9 minutes doing cool-down stretches.

When I get halfway through this program (week 3), my reward to myself will be:

When I complete this program, my reward to myself will be:

Signature: _____

Walking Diary

Week 1

Goal: ___ total minutes or ___ total distance for the week. How did I do each day?

Sunday _____

Monday _____

Tuesday _____

Wednesday _____

Thursday _____

Friday _____

Saturday _____

Starting Point Self-test Pain:_____ Fatigue: _____ Physical Limitations: _____

What's helping me to keep walking?

_____

_____

_____

What's been a challenge for me to keep walking?

_____

_____

_____

What information do I need to help me handle the challenges and where can I get it?

_____

_____

_____

Walking Diary

Week 2

Goal: ___ total minutes or ___ total distance for the week. How did I do each day?

Sunday _____

Monday _____

Tuesday _____

Wednesday _____

Thursday _____

Friday _____

Saturday _____

This week I chose this as my fitness measure:

_____

What's helping me to keep walking?

_____

_____

_____

What's been a challenge for me to keep walking?

_____

_____

_____

What information do I need to help me handle the challenges and where can I get it?

_____

_____

_____

Walking Diary

Week 3

Goal: ___ total minutes or ___ total distance for the week. How did I do each day?

Sunday _____

Monday _____

Tuesday _____

Wednesday _____

Thursday _____

Friday _____

Saturday _____

What's helping me to keep walking?

_____

_____

_____

What's been a challenge for me to keep walking?

_____

_____

_____

What information do I need to help me handle the challenges and where can I get it?

_____

_____

_____

Do I remember to reward myself?

_____

Walking Diary

Week 4

Goal: ___ total minutes or ___ total distance for the week. How did I do each day?

Sunday _____

Monday _____

Tuesday _____

Wednesday _____

Thursday _____

Friday _____

Saturday _____

Now my fitness level is:

_____

What's helping me to keep walking?

_____

_____

_____

What's been a challenge for me to keep walking?

_____

_____

_____

What information do I need to help me handle the challenges and where can I get it?

_____

_____

_____

Walking Diary

Week 5

Goal: ___ total minutes or ___ total distance for the week. How did I do each day?

Sunday _____

Monday _____

Tuesday _____

Wednesday _____

Thursday _____

Friday _____

Saturday _____

What's helping me to keep walking?

_____

_____

_____

What's been a challenge for me to keep walking?

_____

_____

_____

What information do I need to help me handle the challenges and where can I get it?

_____

_____

_____

_____

_____

Walking Diary

Week 6

Goal: ___ total minutes or ___ total distance for the week. How did I do each day?

Sunday _____

Monday _____

Tuesday _____

Wednesday _____

Thursday _____

Friday _____

Saturday _____

Ending Point Self-test Pain:_____ Fatigue: _____ Physical Limitations: _____

Now my fitness level is:

_____

What's helping me to keep walking?

_____

_____

What's been a challenge for me to keep walking?

_____

_____

What information do I need to help me handle the challenges and where can I get it?

_____

_____

Did I remember to reward myself?

_____

Thinking About All Six Weeks

How did I do overall?

_____

_____

_____

_____

_____

_____

What do I want to change?

_____

_____

_____

_____

_____

_____

_____

Other notes:

_____

_____

_____

_____

_____

_____

_____

_____

Appendix B

Exercises to Help You Warm Up, Stretch, and Cool Down

As outlined in the 5-Step Basic Walking Pattern in Chapter 5, after warming up, you should gently stretch, and after cooling down, you should stretch again. This section gives you instructions for warming up, key stretches, additional stretches, and strengthening exercises that will help your walking program.

Ideally, you will go through the 5-Step Basic Walking Pattern each time you walk, even if you walk in 10-minute sessions several times during the day. However, when your time is limited, stretch before and after walking at least one time each day you walk – the first time you walk during the day might make the most sense.

Because you don't want to stretch your muscles when they're cold, be sure to warm up for 3 to 5 minutes first. After you have warmed up, stretch the principle muscle groups for walking: calves, hamstrings, quadriceps and hip flexors, and iliotibial bands. If you are concerned about your balance, do the seated version of the stretches. Hold each stretch for 30 seconds on each side of your body. It should take you no more than 5 minutes to complete your warm-up stretches. After you cool down (3 to 5 minutes), repeat them. This time, hold each stretch for 45 seconds to 1 minute on each side of your body. The cool-down stretches should take from 7 minutes to no more than 9 minutes.

Also included here are some additional warm-up stretches you may wish to try, as well as some strengthening exercises you may wish to do three times a week.

Precautions

By each picture there are notes about precautions you should take.

Balance. Be careful to maintain your balance. Hold on to a stable object (e.g., a chair, railing, wall, or counter) while doing this exercise.

Joint surgery. If you have had recent joint surgery, then check with your doctor before doing this exercise.

Muscle cramps. Stop this exercise if it causes a muscle cramp.

Osteoporosis. If you have osteoporosis or a back compression fracture, then check with your doctor before doing this exercise.

Warm Up Before Stretching

Here are 2 suggestions for warming up:

1. walk slowly for 3 to 5 minutes

2. march in place for 3 to 5 minutes.

Marching in place
PRECAUTIONS: JOINT SURGERY, BALANCE

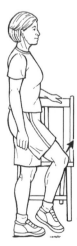

- Stand, holding on to a supportive railing or the back of a chair.

- Hold on to two chairs if you feel unsteady.

- Alternate lifting knees up and down as if marching in place.

- March in place for 3 to 5 minutes.

- Gradually try to lift knees higher and/or march faster toward the end.

Key Stretches To Do
Before and After You Walk

Before you walk, stretch your calf muscles, your hamstrings, your hip flexors and quadriceps, and your iliotibial bands. If you have concerns about your balance, do the seated version of the exercises. Here are some additional hints about stretching:

- Stretch just until you feel tension, and then hold the stretch in that place.

- Stretch gently and smoothly, and do not bounce.

- Be sure to do each stretch on both right and left sides.

- Breathe naturally as you hold the stretches. Don't hold your breath.

1. Stretch your calf muscles.
PRECAUTIONS: JOINT SURGERY, BALANCE

- Lean against a wall, tree, or chair for support.

- Place yout right foot back and keep your toes facing forward.

- Slightly bend the knee of your left leg, never letting your knee go beyond your toes.

- Keep your head up and spine straight.

- Press the heel of your right foot into the ground.

- Hold and then repeat with your left leg.

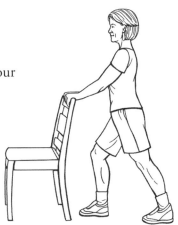

2. Stretch Your Hamstrings – Standing
PRECAUTIONS: MUSCLE CRAMPS, BALANCE

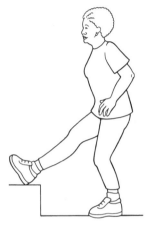

- Holding onto a supportive railing or wall, place your right leg on a slightly raised surface, like a step or a curb.

- Keep your hips facing forward and your standing knee bent.

- Slowly bend your left knee until you feel a very mild tension or stretch on the back of your right thigh.

- To stretch a little more, bend forward just a little at your hips, keeping your back straight.

- Hold and then repeat with your other leg.

Stretch Your Hamstrings – Seated (if concerned about your balance)
PRECAUTION: MUSCLE CRAMPS

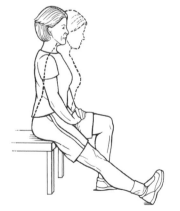

- Sit on the edge of a bench, chair, or other low, firm surface.

- Stretch out your right leg with your toes pointing up, and place your hands on your left thigh.

- Keep your left foot flat on the ground.

- Keeping your back straight, gently lean forward from your hips until you feel a stretch in the back of your right thigh.

- Pull your foot back, pointing your toes up.

- You may feel a stretch by just straightening up your back.

- Hold and then repeat with your left leg.

3. Stretch Your Hip Flexors and Quadriceps – Standing
PRECAUTIONS: JOINT SURGERY, BALANCE

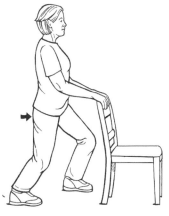

- Step forward with your left foot, keeping your right knee bent.

- Tuck your buttocks tightly under your hips.

- You will feel a stretch on the front of your right hip and upper thigh.

- Hold and then repeat with your left leg.

Seated (if concerned about your balance)
PRECAUTION: JOINT SURGERY

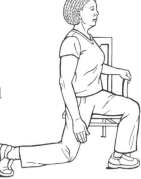

- Sit on the side of a stable chair, bench, or other low firm surface.

- Gently move your right leg back and behind you.

- Tuck your buttocks tightly under your hips.

- You will feel a stretch on the front of your right hip and upper thigh.

- Slide to the opposite side of the chair.

- Repeat with your left leg.

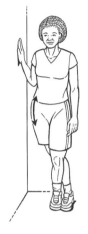

4. Stretch your Iliotibial bands (ITBs)
PRECAUTIONS: JOINT SURGERY, BALANCE

• Stand with your right hip less than foot from a wall.

• Cross your left leg in front, but don't put weight on it, and use your right arm against the wall for support, keeping both knees slightly bent.

• Lean toward the wall with your right hip until you feel a stretch on the outside of your right hip.

• Turn around and repeat on the other side.

Additional Stretches You May Wish to Try

Bent leg calf stretch
PRECAUTIONS: JOINT SURGERY, BALANCE

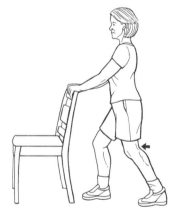

• Lean against a wall, tree, or chair for support.

• Place your right foot back, keeping your toes facing forward.

• Slightly bend your left knee, never letting it go beyond your toes.

• Slightly bend your right knee, as well.

• Keep your head up and spine straight.

• Press the heel of the right foot into the ground.

• Hold and then repeat with the left leg.

Front of calf and toe stretch
PRECAUTIONS: JOINT SURGERY, BALANCE

- Lean against a wall, tree, or chair for support.

- Bend your left knee slightly, never letting it go beyond your toes

- Put your right leg back with the toe pointing straight back.

- Keep your head up and spine straight.

- Gently press front of back foot and lower leg toward floor.

- Hold and then repeat with your left leg.

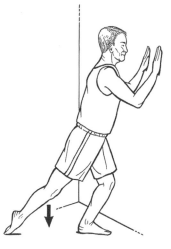

Strengthening Exercises for Walking

Do these exercises three times each week to help strengthen the muscles and joints you use when you walk. Start with 5 to 10 repetitions on each side; increase to no more than 30 repetitions. As for the stretching exercises, if you have concerns about your balance and a seated version is suggested here, do that one. If you have ongoing, severe pain in your knees, ankles, or hips, talk to your health care practitioner to get specific exercise recommendations. Here are some more hints.

- Be sure to do each exercise with both right and left sides.

- Go slowly, and do each movement with control.

- Breathe naturally. Don't hold your breath!

- If you have increased pain that lasts for more than two hours after exercising, next time do fewer repetitions.

Standing back leg lift
PRECAUTIONS: JOINT SURGERY, BALANCE

- Hold on to a counter, table, railing, or wall for support.

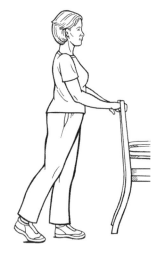

- Stand straight and lift your right foot back (keeping your ankle bent) until only your right toes are on the floor, then bring your foot forward again.

- Keep your right leg straight as you move it back and forth.

- Stand straight and don't lean forward, so the motion comes from your hip and you feel the muscles tightening in your buttocks.

- Return only your toes to the floor between repetitions.

- Repeat with your left foot.

- Repeat 5 times on each side to start, increasing to no more than 30 times on each side.

Heel and toe raises
Standing
PRECAUTIONS: JOINT SURGERY, BALANCE, MUSCLE CRAMPS

- Hold on to a counter, table, railing, or wall for support
- Lift your toes, keeping your heels on the floor.
- Hold for a count of 5.
- Lower slowly.
- Lift your heels, keeping your toes on the floor.
- Hold for a count of 5.
- Lower slowly.
- Repeat 5 times to start, increasing to no more than 30 times.
- It is easier to do both legs at the same time. If your feet are too sore, then wear shoes or do this exercise while sitting down.

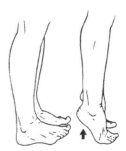

Seated (if concerned about your balance)
PRECAUTIONS: JOINT SURGERY, BALANCE, MUSCLE CRAMPS

- Sit down with or without your shoes on.
- Lift your toes, keeping your heels on the floor.
- Hold for a count of 5.
- Lower slowly
- Lift your heels, keeping your toes on the floor.
- Hold for a count of 5.
- Lower slowly.
- Repeat 5 times to start, increasing to no more than 30 times.
- It is easier to do both legs at the same time

Basic quadriceps strengthening
Standing
PRECAUTION: BALANCE

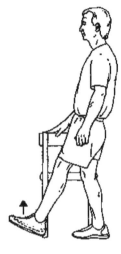

- Hold onto a counter, table railing, or wall for support.

- Stand on your right foot, keeping your right knee slightly bent.

- Bring your left leg forward so it is slightly off the ground, but tighten the muscles on the top of your left thigh before you do it.

- Repeat 5 times to start, increasing to no more than 30 times.

- Repeat standing on your left foot and using your right leg.

Seated (if concerned about your balance)
PRECAUTION: NONE

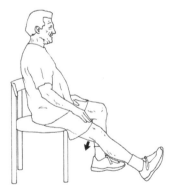

- Sitting on the edge of a chair, put your right leg out in front of you, with it resting on the ground.

- Tighten the muscles on the top of your right thigh by gently pushing the back of your right knee toward the floor.

- Hold for a count of 5.

- Repeat 5 times to start, increasing to no more than 30 times.

- Repeat with your left leg.

Additional quadriceps strengthening, lying on your back
PRECAUTION: OSTEOPOROSIS

- Bend your left knee and place your left foot flat on the bed.
- Tighten the muscle above your right knee, and bend your right ankle.
- Lift your right leg from a few inches to no higher than your left knee.
- Hold for a count of 5.
- Lower slowly.
- Repeat 5 times to start, increasing to no more than 30 times.
- Repeat with your left leg.

If you can easily do this exercise 30 times on each side without pain, you can add a 1- to 2-pound strap ankle weight to each side at a time and do the exercise as described. Start slowly, though, repeating 5 times to start and increasing to no more than 30 on each leg.

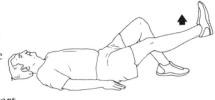

Standing mini-squats
PRECAUTION: BALANCE
(STOP THIS EXERCISE IF IT HURTS YOUR KNEES.)

- Hold onto a counter, table, railing, or wall for support.
- Stand straight with your feet hip distance apart.
- Turn your feet slightly outward.
- Squeeze your buttocks together.
- Slowly bend your knees to lower your body just a few inches.
- Keep your feet flat and do not allow your knees to go past your toes.
- Hold for a count of 5.
- Repeat 5 times to start, increasing to no more than 30 times.

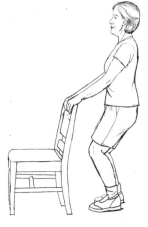

Appendix C

Resources and References

Resources

The Arthritis Foundation

For more than 60 years, the Arthritis Foundation has been the source for reliable information for the nearly 50 million Americans with arthritis. It is the only national, voluntary health organization that works for all people affected by any one of the more than 100 forms of arthritis or related conditions. Local offices nationwide help to support research, professional and community education programs, services for people with arthritis, government advocacy and fundraising activities.

The mission of the Arthritis Foundation is to improve lives through leadership in the prevention, control and cure of arthritis and related diseases. Public contributions and sales of books (like this one) enable the Arthritis Foundation to fulfill this mission, by helping to fund research, programs and services. The Arthritis Foundation has more than 150 local offices all around the United States that provide support for people living with arthritis, including physician referrals, programs and activities, and useful information that helps people with arthritis lead healthier, more fulfilling lives. Arthritis doesn't have to prevent you from doing the activities you enjoy most. While research holds the key to future cures or preventions for arthritis, equally important is improving the quality of life for people with arthritis today.

Information Hotline

The Arthritis Foundation – the expert on arthritis – is only a phone call away. Call toll-free at 1-800-283-7800 for automated information on arthritis and to order free print materials 24 hours a day. Trained volunteers and staff are also available at your local Arthritis Foundation office to answer your questions or send you a list of physicians in your area who specialize in arthritis. Also, choose from our more than 60 educational booklets on different types of arthritis, medications, disease management, self-help and more.

Arthritis Help Online

The Arthritis Foundation's interactive Web site, www.arthritis.org, provides a great deal of information and resources that are easy to access 24 hours a day from your home computer.

Through the Arthritis Foundation Web site, you can chat with other people with arthritis through online message boards, ask questions about your condition and treatment, request free brochures, and purchase books and videos to help you better manage your arthritis. The Arthritis Store contains information about the many books, brochures, and exercise videos published by the Arthritis Foundation. In addition, you can read free material on www.arthritis.org, including in-depth feature stories from *Arthritis Today* magazine and news stories about new research, hot trends, and thought-provoking issues related to arthritis prevention and treatment.

Arthritis Foundation Local Offices

If you have arthritis, your best source of information and support is your local Arthritis Foundation office. The staff at your nearest office has many resources to help you live a healthier, more fulfilling life with arthritis. If you are newly diagnosed with a form of arthritis, contact your chapter to find out what they have to offer you. The Arthritis Foundation Web site can help you find your local Arthritis Foundation office easily, and many local Arthritis Foundation offices have their own Web pages that will inform you about exercise programs, classes, and other events in your community, as well as exciting opportunities to take part in fundraising events, walks, and marathons. Most Arthritis Foundation offices can give you a list of doctors in your area who specialize in the evaluation and treatment of arthritis and arthritis-related diseases.

Exercise Programs and Other Classes

Many people who become involved in one type of physical activity and find that they like it go on to explore other kinds of programs that also are enjoyable and offer health benefits. No matter what your ability, the Arthritis Foundation can help you keep moving. The Arthritis Foundation offers both land- and water-based programs that benefit beginners as well as exercise veterans. Contact your local office to find out where and when these programs will be held.

- The Arthritis Foundation Exercise Program is an eight-week instructor led program. It uses gentle activities to help increase joint flexibility and range of motion and help maintain muscle strength. Exercises are done while sitting, standing, or on the floor. Participants previously enrolled in the program have experienced such benefits as increased functional ability, increased self-care behaviors, decreased pain, and decreased depression.

- The Arthritis Foundation Aquatic Program is a safe, ideal environment for relieving arthritis pain and stiffness. The program is offered at three levels: The Basic Program, The Plus Program, and The Deep-Water Program. These programs can be offered either in sessions of up to 12 weeks in length or ongoing, depending on the facility where the program is offered. The Deep Water Program is for people who have progressed beyond the fitness level accommodated for the basic and plus classes. The gentle activities in warm water, with guidance from a trained instructor, will help you gain strength and flexibility. Participants previously enrolled also enjoyed benefits such as decreased pain and stiffness.

- The Arthritis Foundation Tai Chi Program is designed to improve the quality of life for people with arthritis, using Sun-style Tai Chi, one of the four major recognized styles. This style includes agile steps and exercises that may improve mobility, breathing, and relaxation. The movements don't require deep bending or squatting, which makes it easier and more comfortable to learn.

The program itself consists of 12 movements – 6 basic and 6 advanced – a warm-up and a cool-down. Once participants become familiar with the 12 movements, the program is designed to provide continual challenge by reversing the direction of the movements.

- The Arthritis Self-Management Program helps you learn the skills you need to build your own self-management program that helps you to become an active member of your health care team, work better with your health care providers and handle the day-to-day challenges of your disease. The program includes six weeks of group education designed to complement the care provided by your health care team and allow you to share experiences with others. Past participants of the Arthritis Self-Management Program have experienced such benefits as increased knowledge about their arthritis, increased frequency of exercise and relaxation; increased self-confidence, decreased depression and pain, and fewer physician visits.

Publications and Videos

Arthritis Foundation publications are available by calling 1-800-283-7800, or by logging on to www.arthritis.org and selecting the Store tab.

- **Brochures.** The Arthritis Foundation has an array of free educational brochures on a wide variety of arthritis-related topics, from specific diseases, lifestyle challenges, current medications and more. All brochures are concise and easy to understand and point you to other resources for managing your arthritis.

- *Arthritis Today.* This award-winning magazine brings you up-to-date, reliable information about the latest research and treatment options, diet and nutrition, tips for traveling and making your life with arthritis easier and more rewarding. Subscribe to six issues a year, and find all the information you need to achieve a healthier, more active life with arthritis.

- *Books & DVDs.* In addition to *Walk With Ease*, the Arthritis Foundation publishes a number of books and videos for people with arthritis and for others seeking to create a healthier lifestyle. All Arthritis Foundation materials have been given a thorough medical review by leading physicians and health care professionals, so you can be sure that you are receiving sound information about your health, fitness, and arthritis management. Arthritis Foundation books and videos are available through the Arthritis Foundation Web site and 800 number, and they are also sold in bookstores nationwide.

Other Sources of Information and Support

The Centers for Disease Control and Prevention

The Centers for Disease Control and Prevention (CDC) Arthritis Program is designed to improve the quality of life for people affected by arthritis and other rheumatic conditions by working with states and other partners to increase awareness about appropriate arthritis self-management activities and expanding the reach of programs proven to improve the quality of life for people with arthritis.

- EnhanceFitness (EF) EnhanceFitness (formerly Lifetime Fitness) is an evidence-based, community-delivered exercise program proven to increase strength, boost activity levels, and elevate mood. Certified instructors focus on stretching, flexibility, balance, low-impact aerobics, and strength training exercises. Typically classes meet three times a week for one hour.

- Chronic Disease Self-Management Program (CDSMP) is an effective self-management education program for people with chronic health problems. The program specifically addresses arthritis, diabetes, lung, and heart disease, but teaches skills useful for managing a variety of chronic diseases. This program was developed at Stanford University. CDSMP workshops are held in community settings and meet 2 1/2 hours per week for 6 weeks. Workshops are facilitated by two trained leaders, one or both of whom are not health professionals and who have chronic disease themselves. This program covers topic such as techniques to deal with problems associated with chronic disease, appropriate exercise, appropriate use of medications, communicating effectively with family, friends, and health professionals, nutrition, and, how to evaluate new treatments. Participants who took CDSMP demonstrated significant improvements in exercise, communication with physicians, self-reported general health, health distress, fatigue, disability, and social/role activities limitations.

AARP

AARP (www.aarp.org) is a nonprofit, nonpartisan membership organization for people age 50 and over. AARP is dedicated to enhancing quality of life for all as they age. AARP leads positive social change and delivers value to members through information, advocacy and service. In addition to useful information, AARP sponsors several online programs that support walking as a way of enhancing physical fitness.

* AARP Step Up to Better Health is a free online walking program. Users clip on a step counter and track their steps along one of four famous virtual American trails– Lewis and Clark, Alaska Highway, Highway 50, or the Appalachian Trail.

- AARP Get Fit on Route 66 is a free online physical activity adventure that will inspire users to be more active. Here users convert exercise minutes to miles on a virtual journey along America's most famous highway. The program includes healthy recipes, exercise tips and much more. Visit the Web site at http://www.aarp.org/walking.

The American College of Rheumatology

The American College of Rheumatology (ACR) is an organization of and for physicians, health professionals, and scientists that advances rheumatology through programs of education, research, advocacy and practice support that foster excellence in the care of people with arthritis and rheumatic and musculoskeletal diseases. www.rheumatology.org

Association of Rheumatology Health Professionals

The Association of Rheumatology Health Professionals (ARHP) is a division of the American College of Rheumatology. This professional membership society is made up of non-physician health care professionals specializing in rheumatology, such as advanced practice nurses, nurses, occupational therapists, physical therapists, psychologists, social workers, epidemiologists, physician assistants, educators, clinicians, and researchers. www.rheumatology.org

National Institute of Arthritis and Musculoskeletal and Skin Diseases

The National Institute of Arthritis and Musculoskeletal and Skin Diseases (NIAMS) Web site serves the public, patients and health professionals by providing information, locating other information sources, creating health information materials, and participating in a national Federal database on health information. It provides links to a variety of free, educational brochures on arthritis and other musculoskeletal and skin diseases. www.niams.nih.gov

Reading Important Research

Some people with arthritis like to keep up with the research on arthritis treatment, effective exercise programs, and self-management techniques by reading research articles. In addition to the sources cited here for this book, there are new developments every day. The Arthritis Foundation Web site contains reviews and summaries of the latest research, but you may also want to look for new articles through MedlinePlus, http://medlineplus.gov, a service through the U.S. National Library of Medicine and the National Institutes of Health. It is a Web site devoted entirely to providing trusted and up-to-date health information to both consumers and health professionals. You can even use this site to search for health care practitioners in your area.

Bibliography

American College of Sports Medicine. (1998). Position stand: The recommended quantity and quality of exercise for developing an maintaining cardiorespiratory and muscular fitness and flexibility in healthy adults. *Medicine & Science in Sports & Exercise*, 30(6), 975–991.

American Heart Association. (2007). Target heart rate. Available at www.americanheart.org

Brady, T. J., Kruger, J., Helmick, C. G., Callahan, L. F., & Boutaugh, M. L. (2003). Intervention programs for arthritis and other rheumatic diseases. *Health Education & Behavior*, 30(1), 44–63.

Callahan LF, Mielenz T, Freburger J, Shreffler J, Hootman J, Brady T, Buysse K, Schwartz T. A randomized controlled trial of the people with arthritis can exercise program: symptoms, function, physical activity, and psychosocial outcomes. Arthritis Rheum 2008: Jan 15;59(1):92-101.

Cameron, M. (2003). Thermal agents: Cold and Heat. In M. Bredensteiner, S. Fraser & M. Waldman (Eds.), Physical agents in rehabilitation: From research to practice (pp. 133–184). St. Louis, Mo.: Saunders.

Centers for Disease Control. (Reviewed and updated, May 22, 2007). Physical activity for everyone: Recommendations. Available at www.cdc.gov

Chao, D., Foy, C. G., Farmer, D. (2000). Exercise adherence among older adults: Challenges and strategies. *Controlled Clinical Trials*, 21, 212S–217S.

Coleman, E. A., Buchner, D. M., et al. (1996). The relationship of joint symptoms with exercise performance in older adults. Journal of the American Geriatric Society, 44, 14–21.

Cutt, H., Giles-Corti, B., Knuiman, M., & Burke, V. (2007). Dog ownership, health and physical activity: A critical review of the literature. *Health & Place*, 13(1), 261–272.

deJong, Z., & Vliet Vlieland, T. P. M. (2005). Safety of exercise in patients with rheumatoid arthritis. *Current Opinion in Rheumatology*, 17, 177–182.

Devos-Comby, L., Cronan, T., & Roesch, S. C. (2006). Do exercise and self-management interventions benefit patients with osteoarthritise of the knee? A metaanalytic review. *Journal of Rheumatology*, 33(4), 744–756.

Ettinger, W. H., & Afable, R. F. (1994). Physical disability from knee arthritis: The role of exercise as an intervention. *Medicine & Science in Sports & Exercise*, 26, 1435–1440.

Ettinger, W. H., Burns, R., et al. (1997). A randomized trial comparing aerobic exercise and resistance exercise with a health education program in older adults with knee arthritis: The Fitness Arthritis and Seniors Trial (FAST). *JAMA*, 227, 25–31.

Exercise and Arthritis Special Theme Issue. (1994). *Arthritis Care and Research*, 7, 167–236.

Exercise and Arthritis Special Theme Issue. (2003). *Arthritis Care and Research*, 49, 428–477.

Felson, D. T., Zhang, Y., Anthony, J. M., Naimark, A., & Anderson, J. J. (1992). Weight loss reduces the risk for symptomatic knee osteoarthritis in women: The Framingham Study. *Annals of Internal Medicine*, 116(7), 598–599.

Finckh, A., Iversen, M., & Liang, M. H. (2003). The exercise prescription in rheumatoid arthritis: Primum non nocere. *Arthritis & Rheumatism*, 48(9), 2393–2395.

Gabriel, S. E., Crowson, C. S., & O'Fallon, M. (1999). The epidemiology of rheumatoid arthritis in Rochester, Minnesota, 1955–1985. *Arthritis & Rheumatism*, 42(3), 415–420.

Harkcom, T. A., Lampman, R. M., Banwell, B. F., & Castor, C. W. (1985). Therapeutic value of graded aerobic exercise training in rheumatoid arthritis. *Arthritis & Rheumatism*, 28, 32–39.

Jones, K., Adams, D., Winters-Stone, K., & Burckhardt, C. (2006). A comprehensive review of 46 exercise treatment studies in fibromyalgia (1988–2005). *Health and Quality of Life Outcomes*, 4(1), 67ff.

Kovar, P. A., Allegrante, J. P., & al. (1992). Supervised fitness walking in patients with osteoarthritis of the knee. *Annals of Internal Medicine*, 116, 529–534.

Kramer, H. M., & Curhan, G. (2002). The association between gout and nephrolithiasis: The National Health and

Nutrition Examination Survey III, 1988–1994. *American Journal of Kidney Diseases*, 40(1), 37–42.

Lawrence, R. C., Helmick, C. G., Arnett, F. C., Deyo, R. A., Felson, D. T., Giannini, E. H., et al. (1998). Estimates of the prevalence of arthritis and selected musculoskeletal disorders in the United States. *Arthritis & Rheumatism*, 41(5), 778–799.

Lorig, K., & Holman, H. (1993). Arthritis self-management studies: A twelve year review. *Health Education Quarterly*, 20, 17–28.

Macera, C. A., Hootman, J. M., & Sniezek, J. E. (2003). Major public health benefits of physical activity. *Arthritis & Rheumatism*, 49(1), 190–194.

Mannerkorpi, K., & Iversen, M. (2003). Physical exercise in fibromyalgia and related syndromes. *Best Practice & Research Clinical Rheumatology*, 17(4), 629–647.

Mannerkorpi, K., & Iversen, M. (2005). Exercise in fibromyalgia. *Current Opinion in Rheumatology*, 17(2), 190–194.

McHorney, C. A., Ware, J. E., & Anastasia, R. (1993). The MOS 36-Item Short-Form Health Survey (SF-36): II. Psychometric and clinical tests of validity in measuring physical and mental health constructs. *Medical Care*, 31(3), 247–263.

Messier, S. P., Loeser, R. F., Miller, G. D., Morgan, T. M., Rejeski, W. J., Sevick, M. A., et al. (2004). Exercise and dietary weight loss in overweight and obese older adults with knee osteoarthritis: The Arthritis, Diet, and Activity Promotion Trial. *Arthritis & Rheumatism*, 50, 1501–1510.

Minor, M. A. (1990). Physical activity and management of arthritis. *Annals of Behavioral Medicine*, 13, 117–124.

Minor, M. A. (2004). Impact of exercise on osteoarthritis outcomes. *Journal of Rheumatology*, Supplement, 70, 81–86.

Minor, M. A., Hewett, J. E., & al. (1989). Efficacy on physical conditioning exercise in patients with rheumatoid arthritis and osteoarthritis. *Arthritis & Rheumatism*, 32, 1396–1405.

Minor, M. A., & Sanford, M. K. (1993). Physical interventions in the management of pain in arthritis. *Arthritis Care and Research*, 6, 197–206.

Ottawa Panel. (2004). Ottawa Panel evidence-based clinical practice guidelines for therapeutic exercises in the management of rheumatoid arthritis in adults. *Physical Therapy*, 84(10), 934–972.

Perlman, S. G., Connell, K. J., et al. (1990). Dance-based aerobic exercise for rheumatoid arthritis. *Arthritis Care and Research*, 3, 29–35.

Rippe, J. M., Ward, A., Porcari, J. P., & Freedson, P. S. (1988). Walking for health and fitness. *JAMA*, 259, 2720–2724.

Roddy, E., Zhang, W., Doherty, M., Arden, N. K., Barlow, J., Birrell, F., et al. (2005). Evidence-based recommendations for the role of exercise in the management of osteoarthritis of the hip or knee – The MOVE consensus. *Rheumatology*, 44(1), 67–73.

Schoster, B., Callahan, L. F., Meier, A., Mielenz, T., & DiMartino, L. (2005). Participant satisfaction with the People with Arthritis Can Exercise (PACE) Program: A Qualitative Evaluation. Preventing Chronic Disesase [serial online], 2(3). Available at http://www.cdc.gov

Sharma, L., Dunlop, D. D., & Hayes, K. W. (2004). Is a strong quadriceps muscle bad for a patient with knee osteoarthritis? *Annals of Internal Medicine*, 140, 150.

Stenstrom, C. H., & Minor, M. A. (2003). Evidence for the benefit of aerobic and strengthening exercise in rheumatoid arthritis. *Arthritis & Rheumatism*, 49(3), 428–434.

Stenstrom, C. H., & Minor, M. A. (2003). Evidence for the benefit of aerobic and strengthening exercise in rheumatoid arthritis. *Arthritis & Rheumatism*, 49, 428–434.

Turesson, C., & Mattesonk, E. L. (2007). Cardiovascular risk factors, fitness and physical activity in rheumatic diseases. *Current Opinion in Rheumatology*, 19(2), 190–196.

Visit the Arthritis Foundation Web site at www.arthritis.org or call 1-800-283-7800 to find your nearest Arthritis Foundation office and for access to a wealth of information about living well with arthritis and related conditions.

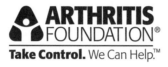

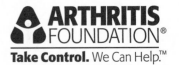

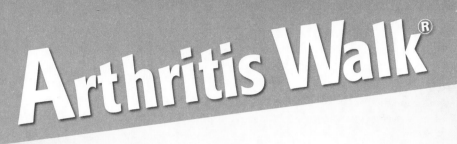
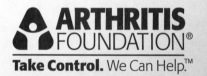